A PERSONALIZED GUIDE TO HEALTH AND FITNESS AFTER 45

(EMPOWER WOMEN TO TAKE CHARGE OF THEIR HEALTH JOURNEY)

By Dr. Angela C Williams

TABLE OF CONTENTS

INTRODUCTION

Greetings and welcome on your journey back to health and vibrancy! If you're reading this, you've taken the first step towards a happier, healthier you.

Let me take you back a few years. It was a typical morning, and like many women juggling multiple roles, I found myself rushing through breakfast while mentally planning the day ahead. As I glanced at my reflection in the mirror, I couldn't help but notice the subtle changes that had crept up over the years. The once-familiar face now bore the marks of time, and my body seemed to carry the weight of responsibilities I had shouldered for so long.

It wasn't just about appearance; it was about how I felt inside. The energy I once took for granted had dwindled, replaced by a sense of fatigue that seemed to linger no matter how much I slept. Simple tasks felt like Herculean feats, and I found myself yearning for the vitality of my younger years.

But amidst the chaos of daily life, I realized something profound: I had the power to change. I could rewrite my story, reclaim my health, and embrace the vibrant life I knew was possible. And so, my journey into weight loss for women over 45 began.

This book isn't just a collection of facts and figures; it's a roadmap to transformation based on real experiences and hard-won lessons. Through my own struggles and triumphs, I've discovered the secrets to sustainable weight loss and renewed vitality, and I'm excited to share them with you.

But before we dive in, I want to extend a heartfelt invitation. I invite you to join me on this journey, to open your mind to new possibilities, and to believe in the power of your own potential. Together, we'll navigate the ups and downs, celebrate victories big and small, and emerge stronger, healthier, and happier than ever before.

Are you prepared to start this experience now? Let's take the first step together and discover the incredible transformation that awaits. Now is the beginning of your path to a happy, healthier you. Let's make it happen!

CHAPTER 1:
WELCOME MESSAGE

Welcome to a journey of transformation and empowerment. As you embark on this path with me, I want to extend my warmest greetings and heartfelt encouragement. Together, we're about to embark on a journey that will not only change our bodies but also transform our lives.

For many years, I struggled with my weight. Like so many women over 45, I found myself facing the daunting challenge of shedding those extra pounds that seemed to stubbornly cling to my body. It wasn't just about fitting into a smaller dress size or conforming to society's standards of beauty. It was about reclaiming my health, my confidence, and my vitality.

I can still clearly recall the important turning point in my journey. It was a crisp autumn morning, and I found myself staring at my reflection in the mirror with a mixture of frustration and determination. I knew that I couldn't continue living in a body that didn't feel like my own. That day, I made a commitment to myself—a commitment to prioritize my health and well-being above all else.

This book is the culmination of that commitment—a testament to the countless hours of research, trial, and error, and ultimately, triumph. Through my own experiences and those of other women just like you, I've distilled the most effective strategies for weight loss and wellness specifically tailored to women over 45.

But before we dive into the nitty-gritty details of nutrition, exercise, and lifestyle changes, I want to take a moment to acknowledge something important: You are not alone. No matter where you are in your journey or how many times you've tried and failed in the past, know that I am here to support you every step of the way.

Together, we will navigate the ups and downs of weight loss with grace and resilience. We will celebrate our successes and learn from our setbacks. And most importantly, we will cultivate a sense of self-love and acceptance that goes far beyond the number on the scale.

I therefore cordially welcome you to go with me on this adventure—a journey of self-realization, empowerment, and metamorphosis. Together, we will unlock the secrets to lasting weight loss and discover the joy of living life to the fullest. Are you ready? Let's begin.

ABOUT THE AUTHOR

Hello there! It's a pleasure to have the opportunity to share a bit about myself with you. My name is Dr. Angela C Williams and I'm honoured to be your guide on this journey toward healthier living.

My passion for health and wellness began long before I ever thought about writing a book. As a young girl, I was always fascinated by the human body—its intricate workings, its resilience, and its capacity for healing. I would spend hours pouring over books and articles, soaking up every bit of information I could find about nutrition, fitness, and holistic well-being.

However, like many women, my own journey toward better health was filled with ups and downs. I struggled with my weight for years, bouncing from one fad diet to the next in search of a quick fix. It wasn't until I reached my mid-40s that I finally realized that true transformation isn't about finding a magic solution—it's about making sustainable lifestyle changes that nourish both body and soul.

Through trial and error, I began to discover what worked for me and what didn't. I experimented with different dietary approaches, explored various forms of exercise, and delved into the world of mindfulness and self-care. Along the way, I encountered setbacks and challenges, but I also experienced moments of profound insight and personal growth.

One of the most valuable lessons I learned on my journey is the importance of listening to my body. Instead of viewing food as the enemy or exercise as a punishment, I learned to cultivate a sense of mindfulness and self-compassion in everything I do. I discovered that true health isn't about restriction or deprivation—it's about nourishing your body with love and respect.

In addition to my personal experiences, I also hold certifications in nutrition, fitness, and wellness coaching. I've spent years studying the latest research and staying up-to-date on the most effective strategies for weight loss and overall well-being. But perhaps most importantly, I bring to this book a deep sense of empathy and understanding for the challenges that women face when it comes to their health.

My goal in writing this book is not to provide a one-size-fits-all solution or to preach from a place of authority. Instead, I hope to empower you to become the CEO of your own health—to take charge of your well-being and make informed choices that align with your unique needs and values.

As we embark on this journey together, know that I am here to support you every step of the way. Whether you're just starting out on your path to better health or you're looking for fresh inspiration to reignite your passion, I am committed to helping you achieve your goals and live your best life.

I appreciate you putting your health and wellbeing in my hands. I am honoured to be a part of your journey, and I can't wait to see all that you will accomplish. Let's make this journey one to remember!

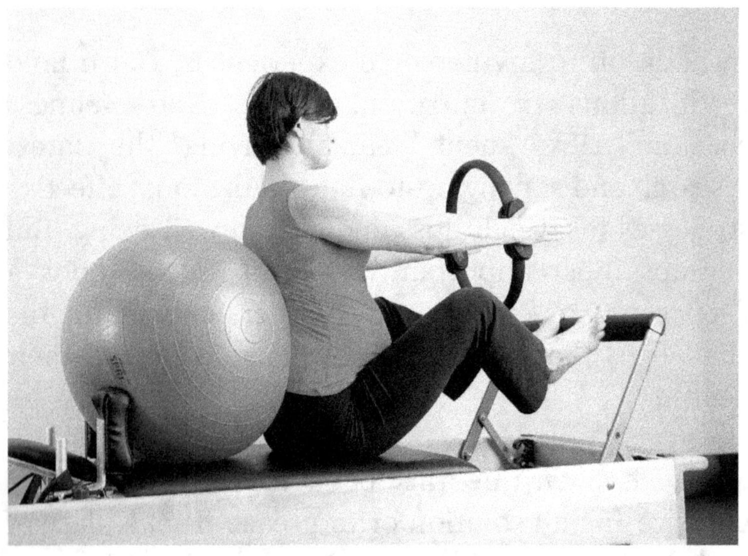

WHY WEIGHT LOSS MATTERS FOR WOMEN OVER 45

Welcome to a crucial discussion about why weight loss is not just a matter of vanity, but a vital component of health and well-being, particularly for women over 45. In this chapter, we'll delve into the specific reasons why maintaining a healthy weight becomes increasingly important as we age, and explore practical tips to address these concerns.

As we reach midlife and beyond, our bodies undergo significant changes that can impact our weight and overall health. Hormonal fluctuations, slowing metabolism, decreased muscle mass, and lifestyle factors all play a role in making weight management more challenging. But why does weight loss matter so much at this stage of life?

1. Health Risks: Excess weight, especially around the midsection, has been linked to an increased risk of various health conditions, including heart disease, type 2 diabetes, high blood pressure, and certain cancers. For women over 45, these risks become even more pronounced, making weight loss a crucial step in reducing the likelihood of developing these serious health issues.

Practical Tip: Focus on adopting a balanced diet rich in whole foods, fruits, vegetables, lean proteins, and healthy fats to support weight loss and overall health. Incorporate regular physical activity into your routine, aiming for a combination of cardio and strength training exercises to boost metabolism and improve body composition.

2. Hormonal Changes: Menopause brings about significant hormonal shifts, including a decline in estrogen levels, which can contribute to weight gain, particularly around the abdomen. This redistribution of fat increases the risk of metabolic syndrome and other related health conditions.

Practical Tip: Pay attention to portion sizes and be mindful of your calorie intake, as metabolism tends to slow down with age. Consider incorporating foods rich in phytoestrogens, such as soy products and flaxseeds, which may help alleviate some menopausal symptoms and support weight management.

3. Bone Health: As women age, bone density naturally decreases, putting them at greater risk of osteoporosis and fractures. Maintaining a healthy weight and engaging in weight-bearing exercises are essential for preserving bone health and reducing the risk of fractures.

Practical Tip: Include calcium-rich foods, such as dairy products, leafy greens, and fortified foods, in your diet to support bone health. Incorporate weight-bearing exercises, such as walking, jogging, or strength training, into your fitness routine to help maintain bone density and prevent osteoporosis.

4. Quality of Life: Carrying excess weight can take a toll on your quality of life, affecting your energy levels, mobility, and overall well-being. By achieving and maintaining a healthy weight, you can enjoy greater vitality, improved mood, and enhanced confidence as you navigate the challenges of ageing.

Practical Tip: Prioritise self-care activities that promote relaxation and stress management, such as meditation, yoga, or deep breathing exercises. Practise mindful eating habits, paying attention to hunger and fullness cues, and savoring each bite to enhance satisfaction and enjoyment of meals.

In conclusion, weight loss matters for women over 45 because it directly impacts their health, vitality, and quality of life. By understanding the specific challenges and risks associated with weight gain during this stage of life, and implementing practical strategies to address them, women can empower themselves to achieve lasting success in their weight loss journey. Remember, it's never too late to take control of your health and embrace a healthier, happier lifestyle.

CHAPTER 2:

UNDERSTANDING WEIGHT LOSS

Welcome to the exploration of understanding weight loss, a journey where we demystify the process and equip ourselves with the knowledge needed to achieve lasting success. In this chapter, we'll break down the fundamentals of weight loss in simple terms, helping you grasp the key principles behind shedding those extra pounds.

1. Basics of Weight Loss:

Weight loss ultimately boils down to a simple equation: calories in versus calories out. When you consume fewer calories than your body needs to maintain its current weight, you create a calorie deficit, prompting your body to burn stored fat for energy, leading to weight loss.

Practical Tip: To create a calorie deficit, focus on making small, sustainable changes to your diet and lifestyle. Start by reducing portion sizes, choosing nutrient-dense foods, and increasing your physical activity levels gradually.

2. Factors Affecting Weight Loss:

While the calorie deficit is the foundation of weight loss, several factors can influence the rate and effectiveness of your efforts. These factors include metabolism, genetics, hormonal balance, age, and lifestyle habits.

Practical Tip: While some factors, such as genetics and age, are beyond your control, you can optimize others to support your weight loss goals. Focus on improving your metabolism through regular exercise, strength training to build lean muscle mass, and prioritizing quality sleep to regulate hormones and support overall health.

3. Understanding Body Composition:

Weight loss is not just about losing pounds on the scale; it's also about improving body composition—the ratio of fat to lean muscle mass in your body. A healthy body composition is essential for overall health and well-being, as excess fat, especially visceral fat around the abdomen, is associated with an increased risk of various health conditions.

Practical Tip: Instead of fixating solely on the number on the scale, pay attention to other indicators of progress, such as measurements, body fat percentage, and how your clothes fit. Aim to incorporate strength training exercises into your routine to build lean muscle mass and improve body composition.

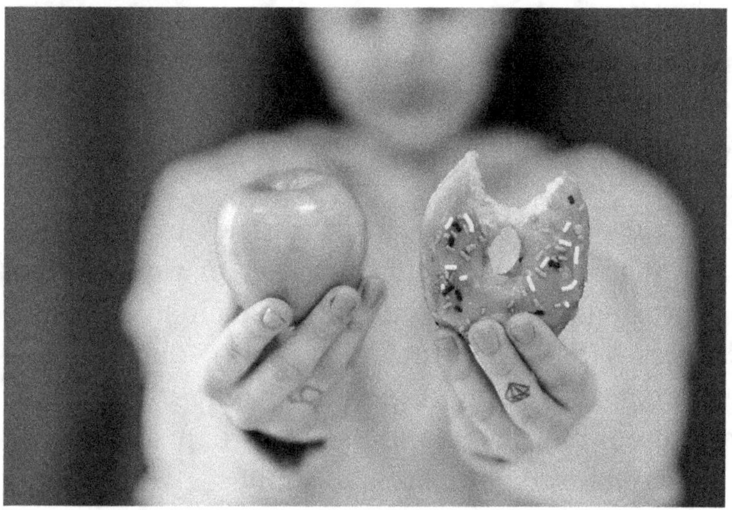

4. Common Misconceptions:

In the quest for weight loss, it's easy to fall prey to common misconceptions and myths perpetuated by the media and diet industry. Understanding these misconceptions can help you separate fact from fiction and make informed choices about your health.

Practical Tip: Be wary of fad diets, quick-fix solutions, and unrealistic promises of rapid weight loss. Instead, focus on adopting sustainable lifestyle changes that promote long-term health and well-being. Consult reputable sources, such as registered dietitians and healthcare professionals, for personalized guidance and support.

In conclusion, understanding weight loss is essential for laying the foundation of a successful journey toward a healthier, happier you. By grasping the basics of how weight loss works, recognizing the factors that influence it, and dispelling common misconceptions, you can empower yourself to make informed choices and achieve lasting results. Remember, weight loss is not a one-size-fits-all approach—find what works best for you and embrace the journey with patience, perseverance, and positivity.

BASICS OF WEIGHT LOSS

Welcome to the foundation of your weight loss journey—understanding the basics of how weight loss works and how you can achieve your goals effectively and sustainably. In this chapter, we'll delve into the fundamental principles of weight loss, drawing from both scientific knowledge and personal experiences to guide you on your path to success.

My journey with weight loss began with a simple realisation: it's not about following restrictive diets or punishing myself with gruelling workouts. Instead, it's about understanding the basic principles of how our bodies process food and energy, and making informed choices that support our health and well-being.

1. Calories In, Calories Out:

At its core, weight loss comes down to a basic equation: calories in versus calories out. When you consume more calories than your body needs to maintain its current weight, the excess calories are stored as fat, leading to weight gain. Conversely, when you consume fewer calories than your body needs, you create a calorie deficit, prompting your body to burn stored fat for energy, resulting in weight loss.

To put it simply, if you consistently consume fewer calories than your body expends, you will lose weight over time. However, it's important to strike a balance and avoid extremes, as overly restrictive diets or excessive calorie deficits can be unsustainable and detrimental to your health.

2. Quality of Calories:

While calorie balance is important for weight loss, the quality of the calories you consume also plays a significant role in your overall health and well-being. Not all calories are created equal—foods that are high in nutrients, such as fruits, vegetables, lean proteins, and whole grains, provide essential vitamins, minerals, and fibre that support optimal health.

On the other hand, foods that are high in added sugars, refined carbohydrates, and unhealthy fats can contribute to weight gain and increase the risk of various health conditions, such as heart disease, type 2 diabetes, and inflammation.

3. Portion Control:

In addition to focusing on the quality of your calories, practicing portion control is key to managing your calorie intake and achieving your weight loss goals. It's easy to underestimate portion sizes, especially in a culture where oversized portions have become the norm.

One effective strategy for portion control is to use visual cues, such as the palm of your hand or a deck of cards, to estimate appropriate serving sizes. Another helpful tip is to pay attention to hunger and fullness cues, eating mindfully and stopping when you feel satisfied, rather than stuffed.

4. Mindful Eating:

Mindful eating is a practice that involves paying attention to the sensory experience of eating, including the taste, texture, and aroma of food, as well as your hunger and fullness cues. By slowing down and savouring each bite, you can enhance your enjoyment of food, prevent overeating, and foster a healthier relationship with food.

One way to incorporate mindful eating into your routine is to eliminate distractions, such as television or smartphones, during meals, and focus solely on the act of eating. Take the time to chew your food slowly, savouring the flavours, and pausing between bites to check in with your body's hunger and fullness signals.

In conclusion, the basics of weight loss are rooted in simple yet powerful principles: create a calorie deficit, focus on the quality of your calories, practice portion control, and embrace mindful eating. By understanding these fundamentals and applying them to your daily life, you can achieve lasting success on your weight loss journey. Remember, progress may be gradual, but every small step you take brings you closer to your goals.

COMMON MISCONCEPTIONS ABOUT WEIGHT LOSS

Welcome to a chapter dedicated to unraveling the myths and misunderstandings surrounding weight loss. In this section, we'll address some of the most prevalent misconceptions that often lead to frustration and confusion on the journey to achieving a healthier weight. Let's get started and distinguish reality from fiction.

1. Myth: You Must Avoid Carbohydrates to Lose Weight

One of the most widespread misconceptions about weight loss is the belief that carbohydrates are inherently bad and must be avoided to shed pounds. While it's true that some carbohydrates, such as sugary snacks and refined grains, can contribute to weight gain when consumed in excess, not all carbs are created equal.

Reality: Carbohydrates are an essential source of energy for our bodies, particularly for activities requiring quick bursts of energy, such as high-intensity exercise. The key is to focus on consuming complex carbohydrates from whole, unprocessed sources, such as fruits, vegetables, legumes, and whole grains, which provide essential nutrients and fiber to support overall health and satiety.

Practical Tip: Instead of demonising all carbohydrates, aim to make healthier choices by prioritising whole, nutrient-dense sources over refined and processed options. Incorporate a variety of colourful fruits and vegetables into your meals, choose whole grains like quinoa, brown rice, and oats, and opt for fibre-rich legumes such as beans and lentils to keep you feeling full and satisfied.

2. Myth: You Can Lose Weight Quickly and Easily with a Fad Diet

In our fast-paced society, the allure of quick-fix solutions for weight loss is undeniable. From juice cleanses to extreme low-calorie diets, fad diets promise rapid results with minimal effort, but at what cost?

Reality: While fad diets may lead to short-term weight loss, they are often unsustainable and can have harmful effects on your physical and mental health. These diets typically restrict certain food groups, severely limit calorie intake, or rely on expensive supplements or meal replacements, making them difficult to maintain in the long run. Additionally, rapid weight loss can result in muscle loss, nutrient deficiencies, and a slowed metabolism, making it harder to maintain weight loss over time.

Practical Tip: Instead of falling for the allure of quick-fix diets, focus on making gradual, sustainable changes to your eating habits and lifestyle. Adopt a balanced approach to nutrition, including a variety of whole foods from all food groups, and aim for slow, steady progress rather than rapid weight loss. Consult with a registered dietitian or healthcare professional for personalised guidance and support in developing a healthy eating plan that meets your individual needs and preferences.

3. Myth: Exercise Alone is Sufficient for Weight Loss

While exercise is an important component of a healthy lifestyle and can contribute to weight loss, it's not the sole factor determining success on the scale.

Reality: Weight loss is primarily influenced by the balance between calories consumed and calories expended, with diet playing a more significant role than exercise. While physical activity can help increase calorie expenditure, build lean muscle mass, and improve overall health and fitness, it's essential to accompany exercise with dietary changes to achieve sustainable weight loss.

Practical Tip: Incorporate a combination of cardiovascular exercise, strength training, and flexibility exercises into your weekly routine to maximize calorie burn, build muscle, and improve overall fitness. However, remember that you can't out-exercise a poor diet, so prioritize healthy eating habits alongside regular physical activity for optimal weight loss results.

4. Myth: You Have to Eat Less to Lose Weight

It's a common misconception that weight loss requires strict calorie restriction and constant hunger. However, this approach is neither sustainable nor healthy in the long run.

Reality: While creating a calorie deficit is essential for weight loss, excessively restricting calories can slow down your metabolism, trigger cravings, and lead to nutrient deficiencies. Instead of focusing solely on eating less, aim to eat smarter by choosing nutrient-dense foods that provide satiety and satisfaction without excess calories.

Practical Tip: Focus on filling your plate with whole, minimally processed foods that are rich in nutrients and fibre, such as fruits, vegetables, lean proteins, and whole grains. Prioritise portion control and mindful eating, paying attention to hunger and fullness cues, and stopping when you feel satisfied rather than overly full. By focusing on the quality of your calories and listening to your body's signals, you can achieve sustainable weight loss without resorting to extreme calorie restriction.

In conclusion, debunking common misconceptions about weight loss is essential for setting realistic expectations and making informed choices on your journey to a healthier, happier you. By understanding the truth behind these myths and adopting evidence-based strategies, you can empower yourself to achieve lasting success in your weight loss goals. Remember, there's no one-size-fits-all approach to weight loss—find what works best for you and embrace the journey with patience, persistence, and positivity.

FACTORS AFFECTING WEIGHT LOSS IN WOMEN OVER 45

Welcome to an exploration of the unique factors that can influence weight loss in women over the age of 45. As we journey through midlife and beyond, our bodies undergo various changes that can impact our metabolism, hormone levels, and overall health. Understanding these factors is essential for developing effective strategies to achieve and maintain a healthy weight. Let's delve into some key considerations and practical tips for navigating the challenges of weight loss in this demographic.

1. Hormonal Changes:

One of the most significant factors affecting weight loss in women over 45 is hormonal fluctuations, particularly during perimenopause and menopause. As estrogen levels decline, women may experience changes in metabolism, increased fat storage, and redistribution of body fat, often leading to weight gain, especially around the abdomen.

Practical Tip: To mitigate the effects of hormonal changes on weight gain, focus on adopting a balanced diet rich in whole foods, fruits, vegetables, lean proteins, and healthy fats. Incorporate regular physical activity into your routine, including both cardiovascular exercise and strength training, to boost metabolism, maintain muscle mass, and support overall health.

2. Slowing Metabolism:

Metabolism naturally slows down with age, primarily due to a loss of muscle mass and a decrease in physical activity levels. As a result, women over 45 may find it more challenging to lose weight and maintain a healthy body composition.

Practical Tip: To combat a slowing metabolism, incorporate strength training exercises into your fitness routine to build and preserve lean muscle mass. Muscle tissue burns more calories at rest than fat tissue, so increasing muscle mass can help boost metabolism and support weight loss efforts. Additionally, engage in regular cardiovascular exercise to increase calorie burn and improve overall fitness.

3. Lifestyle Factors:

Lifestyle factors, such as diet, physical activity, sleep, stress levels, and overall health, can significantly impact weight loss success in women over 45. Busy schedules, caregiving responsibilities, work commitments, and other life stressors can make it challenging to prioritize self-care and make healthy choices.

Practical Tip: Take a holistic approach to weight loss by addressing lifestyle factors that may be hindering your progress. Make self-care a priority by carving out time for regular exercise, adequate sleep, stress management techniques, and relaxation activities. Prioritize nutrient-dense foods and mindful eating habits, and seek support from friends, family, or healthcare professionals to help you stay on track and overcome obstacles.

4. Body Composition Changes:

As women age, changes in body composition, such as a decrease in muscle mass and an increase in body fat percentage, can impact metabolism, energy expenditure, and overall health. Maintaining a healthy body weight and losing weight may become more difficult as a result of these changes.

Practical Tip: Focus on maintaining and building lean muscle mass through regular strength training exercises. Incorporate a combination of resistance exercises, such as weightlifting, bodyweight exercises, and resistance bands, to target major muscle groups and improve overall body composition. Additionally, prioritize protein-rich foods in your diet to support muscle growth and repair.

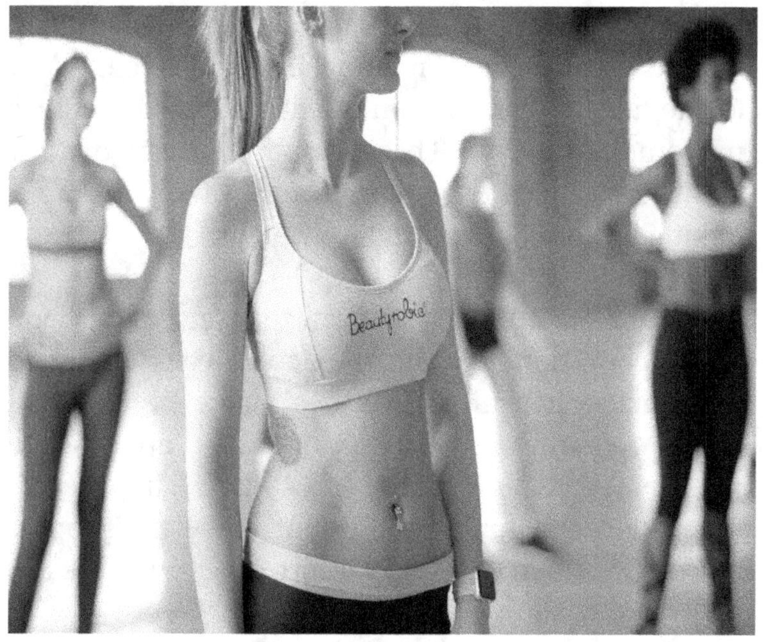

5. Health Conditions:

Certain health conditions, such as thyroid disorders, insulin resistance, metabolic syndrome, and hormonal imbalances, can affect weight loss efforts in women over 45. These conditions can disrupt metabolism, hormone levels, and energy balance, making it more difficult to lose weight.

Practical Tip: If you suspect that an underlying health condition may be impacting your ability to lose weight, consult with a healthcare professional for a thorough evaluation and appropriate management. Addressing any underlying health issues and optimizing treatment can help support weight loss efforts and improve overall health outcomes.

In conclusion, understanding the factors that can affect weight loss in women over 45 is essential for developing effective strategies to achieve and maintain a healthy weight. By addressing hormonal changes, slowing metabolism, lifestyle factors, body composition changes, and underlying health conditions, women can empower themselves to make informed choices and overcome obstacles on their weight loss journey. Remember, progress may be gradual, but with patience, persistence, and dedication, achieving a healthier, happier lifestyle is within reach.

CHAPTER 3:
THE PHYSIOLOGY OF WOMEN OVER 45

Welcome to a chapter dedicated to exploring the unique physiological changes that occur in women over the age of 45. As we navigate through midlife and beyond, our bodies undergo various transformations that can impact our health, vitality, and overall well-being. In this chapter, we'll delve into the intricacies of female physiology at this stage of life, drawing from both scientific knowledge and personal experiences to shed light on this important topic.

1. Hormonal Changes:

One of the hallmark features of female physiology during midlife is hormonal fluctuations, particularly during perimenopause and menopause. As estrogen levels decline and reproductive function wanes, women may experience a range of symptoms, including hot flashes, night sweats, mood swings, and changes in menstrual cycles.

Personal Experience: Like many women in their mid-40s, I found myself grappling with the onset of perimenopause—a time of uncertainty and transition. The sudden appearance of hot flashes and mood swings took me by surprise, leaving me feeling out of control and frustrated. However, through education and support, I learned to navigate this phase with grace and resilience.

Understanding these hormonal changes is crucial for managing symptoms and optimising health during this transitional period. While hormone replacement therapy (HRT) may offer relief for some women, lifestyle modifications, such as regular exercise, stress management, and a balanced diet, can also help alleviate symptoms and support overall well-being.

2. Metabolic Changes:

Another key aspect of female physiology over 45 is metabolic changes, including a slowing metabolism and changes in body composition. As we age, our metabolic rate naturally declines, primarily due to a loss of muscle mass and a decrease in physical activity levels.

Personal Experience: As I entered my late 40s, I noticed that it became increasingly challenging to maintain my weight despite my best efforts. My once reliable metabolism seemed to have hit a plateau, leaving me feeling frustrated and discouraged.

However, by incorporating strength training exercises into my routine and making mindful dietary choices, I was able to revitalise my metabolism and achieve sustainable weight loss.

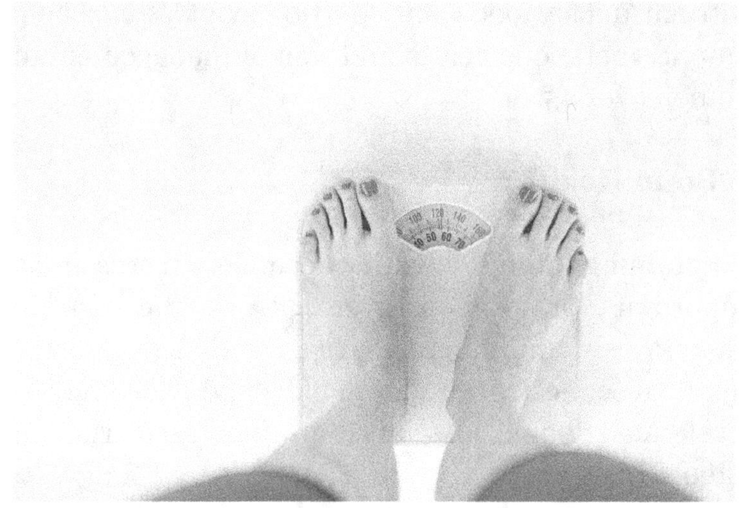

To counteract these metabolic changes, it's essential to prioritise regular physical activity, particularly strength training exercises that build and preserve lean muscle mass. Additionally, focusing on nutrient-dense foods and portion control can help support metabolic health and weight management in women over 45.

3. Bone Health:

Maintaining bone health becomes increasingly important for women over 45, as the risk of osteoporosis and fractures rises with age. During menopause, estrogen levels decline, leading to accelerated bone loss and an increased risk of osteoporosis.

Personal Experience: The fear of osteoporosis loomed large in my mind as I approached my 50s, prompting me to take proactive steps to protect my bone health. Through weight-bearing exercises, such as walking, jogging, and strength training, as well as ensuring an adequate intake of calcium and vitamin D, I was able to strengthen my bones and reduce my risk of fractures.

To support bone health, women over 45 should focus on incorporating calcium-rich foods, such as dairy products, leafy greens, and fortified foods, into their diet. Additionally, engaging in regular weight-bearing exercises and participating in activities that promote balance and coordination can help reduce the risk of falls and fractures.

4. Cardiovascular Health:

Cardiovascular health becomes increasingly important for women over 45, as the risk of heart disease rises with age. Estrogen plays a protective role in cardiovascular health, so as estrogen levels decline during menopause, women become more susceptible to heart disease.

Personal Experience: The realisation of my increased risk of heart disease was a wake-up call for me, prompting me to prioritise cardiovascular health in my daily life. By adopting a heart-healthy diet, engaging in regular exercise, and managing stress effectively, I was able to reduce my risk factors and improve my overall cardiovascular health.

To support cardiovascular health, women over 45 should focus on maintaining a healthy lifestyle that includes regular exercise, a balanced diet, stress management techniques, and regular check-ups with a healthcare professional. By addressing modifiable risk factors, such as high blood pressure, high cholesterol, and smoking, women can reduce their risk of heart disease and improve their overall quality of life.

In conclusion, understanding the physiology of women over 45 is essential for navigating the unique challenges and opportunities of this life stage. By acknowledging and embracing these changes, women can empower themselves to make informed choices that support their health, vitality, and overall well-being. Remember, every woman's journey is unique, so listen to your body, seek support when needed, and embrace the beauty and resilience of the female body at every age.

HORMONAL CHANGES AND WEIGHT GAIN

Welcome to a chapter dedicated to exploring the complex relationship between hormonal changes and weight gain, particularly in women. Hormones play a crucial role in regulating metabolism, appetite, and fat storage, and fluctuations in hormone levels can significantly impact body weight and composition. In this chapter, we'll delve into the hormonal changes that commonly occur in women and how they can contribute to weight gain. Additionally, we'll provide practical tips for managing hormonal imbalances and supporting healthy weight management.

1. Understanding Hormonal Changes:

Hormonal changes are a natural part of life for women, occurring during various stages such as puberty, menstruation, pregnancy, and menopause. These changes are driven by fluctuations in estrogen, progesterone, testosterone, thyroid hormones, insulin, cortisol, and other hormones.

During puberty, hormonal changes can lead to increased appetite and changes in body composition as girls experience growth spurts and changes in fat distribution. Similarly, hormonal fluctuations during the menstrual cycle can cause changes in water retention, cravings, and energy levels.

The most significant hormonal changes for women occur during menopause, typically between the ages of 45 and 55. During this time, estrogen levels decline, leading to symptoms such as hot flashes, night sweats, mood swings, and changes in metabolism. The decrease in estrogen also contributes to changes in fat distribution, with many women experiencing weight gain, particularly around the abdomen.

2. How Hormonal Changes Contribute to Weight Gain:

Several mechanisms can explain how hormonal changes contribute to weight gain in women:

a. Metabolic Changes: Estrogen plays a role in regulating metabolism, and as estrogen levels decline during menopause, metabolism slows down. This can lead to fewer calories burned at rest, making it easier to gain weight, especially if dietary and activity levels remain the same.

b. Appetite Regulation: Hormonal fluctuations can impact appetite regulation, leading to increased hunger and cravings, particularly for high-calorie, high-carbohydrate foods. This can result in overeating and weight gain, especially if not balanced with physical activity.

c. Fat Storage: Estrogen influences where fat is stored in the body, with lower estrogen levels associated with increased fat storage around the abdomen, known as visceral fat. Visceral fat is metabolically active and has been linked to an increased risk of chronic diseases such as heart disease, type 2 diabetes, and certain cancers.

d. Insulin Sensitivity: Changes in hormone levels can affect insulin sensitivity, leading to insulin resistance and increased fat storage, particularly around the abdomen. A risk factor for weight gain and metabolic diseases is insulin resistance.

3. Practical Tips for Managing Hormonal Changes and Weight Gain:

While hormonal changes are a natural part of life for women, there are several practical strategies that can help manage weight gain associated with these changes:

a. Balanced Diet: Focus on a balanced diet rich in whole, nutrient-dense foods such as fruits, vegetables, lean proteins, whole grains, and healthy fats. Avoid excessive consumption of processed foods, sugary snacks, and refined carbohydrates, which can contribute to weight gain and hormonal imbalances.

b. Regular Exercise: Engage in regular physical activity to support metabolism, maintain muscle mass, and manage weight. Aim for a combination of aerobic exercise, strength training, and flexibility exercises to achieve optimal health benefits.

c. Stress Management: Chronic stress can disrupt hormone balance and contribute to weight gain, particularly around the abdomen. Practice stress management techniques such as meditation, yoga, deep breathing exercises, and spending time outdoors to reduce stress levels and support hormonal balance.

d. Adequate Sleep: Prioritise adequate sleep, aiming for seven to nine hours per night, to support hormone regulation, metabolism, and overall health. Poor sleep quality or insufficient sleep can disrupt hormone levels, increase appetite, and contribute to weight gain.

e. Hormone Replacement Therapy (HRT): For women experiencing severe symptoms of menopause, such as hot flashes, night sweats, and mood swings, hormone replacement therapy (HRT) may be recommended to alleviate symptoms and support overall well-being. Nevertheless, it's essential to discuss the possibility of risks and benefits of HRT with a healthcare professional

f. Consultation with Healthcare Provider: If you're experiencing significant weight gain or other symptoms of hormonal imbalance, consult with a healthcare provider for a comprehensive evaluation and personalized treatment plan. Your healthcare provider can conduct hormone tests, assess your overall health, and recommend appropriate interventions to support hormonal balance and weight management.

In conclusion, hormonal changes can significantly impact weight gain in women, particularly during stages such as puberty, menstruation, pregnancy, and menopause. By understanding how hormones influence metabolism, appetite regulation, fat storage, and insulin sensitivity, women can take proactive steps to manage weight gain and support overall health. By adopting a balanced diet, engaging in regular exercise, practising stress management techniques, prioritising sleep, considering hormone replacement therapy if needed, and consulting with a healthcare provider, women can navigate hormonal changes with greater ease and achieve a healthier weight and lifestyle. Remember, every woman's journey is unique, so listen to your body, seek support when needed, and embrace the beauty and resilience of the female body at every stage of life.

METABOLISM AND AGING

Welcome to a chapter dedicated to exploring the fascinating relationship between metabolism and aging. As we journey through life, our metabolism—the process by which our bodies convert food and drink into energy—undergoes changes that can influence our weight, energy levels, and overall health. In this chapter, we'll delve into how metabolism evolves as we age, and provide practical tips for supporting a healthy metabolism throughout the aging process.

Understanding Metabolism:

Metabolism encompasses all the biochemical processes that occur within the body to sustain life. These processes include digestion, absorption, transportation, and utilization of nutrients, as well as the elimination of waste products. At its core, metabolism serves two primary functions: anabolism, which involves building and storing energy, and catabolism, which involves breaking down energy for use by the body.

Metabolism is influenced by various factors, including age, genetics, body composition, hormone levels, activity level, and diet. While some of these factors are beyond our control, others can be modified through lifestyle choices to support a healthy metabolism and overall well-being.

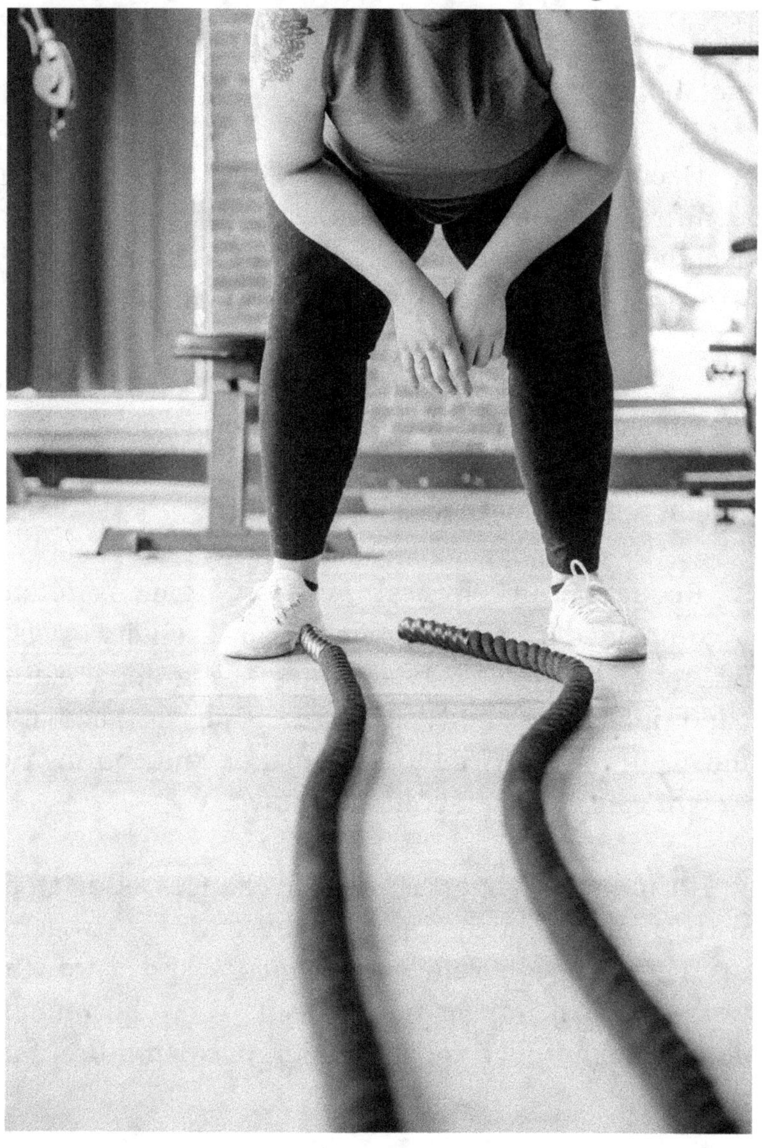

METABOLISM AND AGING :

As we age, several factors contribute to changes in metabolism:

1. Decline in Muscle Mass: One of the most significant changes in metabolism with aging is the decline in muscle mass, known as sarcopenia. Because muscle tissue has a higher metabolic activity than fat tissue, it expels more calories when at rest. As we lose muscle mass with age, our basal metabolic rate—the number of calories our bodies burn at rest—decreases, making it easier to gain weight and harder to lose it.

2. Reduction in Physical Activity: Aging is often accompanied by a decrease in physical activity levels, whether due to lifestyle changes, chronic health conditions, or mobility issues. Less physical activity means fewer calories burned, further contributing to weight gain and metabolic slowdown.

3. Hormonal Changes: Hormonal changes associated with aging, such as declines in estrogen, testosterone, thyroid hormones, and growth hormone, can impact metabolism. These hormonal changes can affect appetite, energy expenditure, fat

storage, and muscle mass, all of which influence metabolism and weight management.

4. Changes in Digestion and Absorption: Aging can also affect digestion and absorption of nutrients, leading to nutrient deficiencies and alterations in metabolism. Digestive enzyme production may decline, stomach acid levels may decrease, and absorption of certain nutrients, such as vitamin B12 and calcium, may become less efficient.

Practical Tips for Supporting a Healthy Metabolism:

While metabolism naturally slows down with age, there are several practical strategies that can help support a healthy metabolism and overall well-being:

1. Stay Active: Engage in regular physical activity, including aerobic exercise, strength training, flexibility exercises, and balance exercises, to support muscle mass, metabolism, and overall health. Aim for at least 150 minutes of moderate-intensity aerobic activity or 75 minutes of vigorous-intensity aerobic activity per week, as well as muscle-strengthening activities on two or more days per week.

2. Maintain Muscle Mass: Incorporate strength training exercises into your fitness routine to build and preserve muscle mass, which can help boost metabolism and support weight management. Focus on compound exercises that target multiple muscle groups, such as squats, lunges, push-ups, and rows, and progressively increase the intensity and volume of your workouts over time.

3. Eat a Balanced Diet: Focus on a balanced diet that includes a variety of nutrient-dense foods such as fruits, vegetables, whole grains, lean proteins, and healthy fats. Prioritize protein-rich foods to support muscle mass, and include sources of omega-3 fatty acids, fiber, vitamins, and minerals to support overall health and metabolism.

4. Watch Portion Sizes: Be mindful of portion sizes and avoid overeating, particularly of high-calorie, high-fat, and processed foods. Pay attention to hunger and fullness cues, and practice mindful eating by eating slowly, savoring each bite, and stopping when you feel satisfied rather than overly full.

5. Stay Hydrated: Drink plenty of water throughout the day to support hydration, digestion, metabolism, and overall health. Aim for at least 8-10 cups of water per day, or more if you're physically active or in a hot climate.

6. Get Adequate Sleep: Prioritize adequate sleep, aiming for 7-9 hours of quality sleep per night, to support metabolism, hormone regulation, and overall health. Poor sleep quality or insufficient sleep can disrupt metabolism, increase appetite, and contribute to weight gain.

7. Manage Stress: Practice stress management techniques such as meditation, deep breathing exercises, yoga, tai chi, and spending time in nature to reduce stress levels and support metabolic health. Chronic stress can disrupt hormone balance, increase cortisol levels, and negatively impact metabolism.

8. Consider Hormone Therapy: If you're experiencing significant hormonal changes or symptoms associated with menopause or other hormonal imbalances, consider discussing hormone replacement therapy (HRT) with a healthcare provider. HRT may help alleviate symptoms and support hormonal balance, but it's essential to weigh the potential risks and benefits and explore alternative treatments as well.

In conclusion, while metabolism naturally slows down with age, there are several practical strategies that can help support a healthy metabolism and overall well-being. By staying active, maintaining muscle mass, eating a balanced diet, watching portion sizes, staying hydrated, getting adequate sleep, managing stress, and considering hormone therapy if needed, you can support your metabolism and thrive at any age. Remember, every small step you take toward supporting your metabolism and overall health can have a positive impact on your quality of life and longevity.

UNDERSTANDING BODY COMPOSITION

Welcome to a chapter dedicated to unravelling the concept of body composition.The percentage of fat, muscle, bone, and other tissues that comprise our bodies is referred to as our body composition. It plays a crucial role in determining overall health, fitness, and well-being. In this chapter, we'll delve into the importance of understanding body composition, how it's measured, and practical tips for optimising body composition for better health.

Why Body Composition Matters:

Body composition is more than just a number on the scale—it provides valuable insights into our health and fitness levels. While weight alone can't distinguish between fat mass and lean mass, body composition analysis allows us to differentiate between the two and assess our overall body composition.

Understanding body composition is essential for several reasons:

1. Health: Excess body fat, particularly visceral fat stored around the abdomen, is associated with an

increased risk of chronic diseases such as heart disease, type 2 diabetes, and certain cancers. By measuring body composition, we can identify areas of excess fat accumulation and take steps to reduce our risk of these diseases.

2. Fitness: Lean muscle mass plays a vital role in metabolism, strength, and functional capacity. By optimizing muscle mass and reducing body fat, we can improve our fitness levels, enhance athletic performance, and reduce the risk of injury.

3. Weight Management: Focusing solely on weight loss can be misleading, as it doesn't necessarily reflect changes in body composition. By monitoring changes in body fat percentage and lean muscle mass, we can track progress more accurately and make adjustments to our diet and exercise routine as needed.

4. Body Image: Understanding body composition can also influence our perception of body image and self-esteem. By focusing on building a healthy body composition rather than achieving a specific weight or size, we can cultivate a more positive relationship with our bodies and prioritise health over appearance.

How Body Composition is Measured:

Several methods can be used to measure body composition, each with its advantages and limitations:

1. Body Mass Index (BMI): BMI is a commonly used measure of body composition that calculates weight in relation to height. While BMI provides a general indication of body fatness, it doesn't differentiate between fat mass and lean mass, and it may not accurately reflect body composition in athletes or individuals with high muscle mass.

2. Waist Circumference: Waist circumference is a simple measure of abdominal fat accumulation and is often used as an indicator of visceral fat and abdominal obesity. A waist circumference greater than 35 inches for women and 40 inches for men is associated with an increased risk of chronic diseases.

3. Dual-Energy X-ray Absorptiometry (DEXA): DEXA is considered the gold standard for measuring body composition, as it provides accurate measurements of bone density, fat mass, and lean muscle mass. However, DEXA scans can be costly and require specialized equipment, making them less accessible for routine use.

4. Bioelectrical Impedance Analysis (BIA): BIA measures body composition by sending a low-level electrical current through the body and analysing the impedance (resistance) encountered by the current. BIA devices are portable, affordable, and non-invasive, making them suitable for home use. However, BIA may not be as accurate as other methods, particularly in individuals with dehydration or certain medical conditions.

Practical Tips for Optimising Body Composition:

Regardless of the method used to measure body composition, there are several practical strategies that can help optimize body composition for better health:

1. Strength Training: Incorporate strength training exercises into your fitness routine to build and preserve lean muscle mass. Focus on compound exercises that target multiple muscle groups, such as squats, deadlifts, lunges, push-ups, and rows. Aim for at least two to three strength training sessions per week, progressively increasing the intensity and volume of your workouts over time.

2. Cardiovascular Exercise: Engage in regular cardiovascular exercise to burn calories, improve cardiovascular health, and support weight

management. Include a variety of activities such as walking, jogging, cycling, swimming, and dancing to keep your workouts fun and engaging. Aim for at least 150 minutes of moderate-intensity aerobic activity or 75 minutes of vigorous-intensity aerobic activity per week, as well as muscle-strengthening activities on two or more days per week.

3. Balanced Diet: Focus on a balanced diet that includes a variety of nutrient-dense foods such as fruits, vegetables, whole grains, lean proteins, and healthy fats. Prioritise protein-rich foods to support muscle growth and repair, and include sources of omega-3 fatty acids, fiber, vitamins, and minerals to support overall health and metabolism. Be mindful of portion sizes and avoid overeating, particularly of high-calorie, high-fat, and processed foods.

4. Hydration: Throughout the day, make sure you drink lots of water to stay hydrated. Adequate hydration supports digestion, metabolism, and overall health, and can help optimise body composition. Aim for at least 8-10 cups of water per day, or more if you're physically active or in a hot climate.

5. Sleep: Prioritise adequate sleep, aiming for 7-9 hours of quality sleep per night, to support metabolism, hormone regulation, and overall health. Poor sleep quality or insufficient sleep can disrupt

metabolism, increase appetite, and contribute to weight gain.

6. Stress Management: Practice stress management techniques such as meditation, deep breathing exercises, yoga, tai chi, and spending time in nature to reduce stress levels and support metabolic health. Chronic stress can disrupt hormone balance, increase cortisol levels, and negatively impact body composition.

7. Monitor Progress: Track changes in body composition over time using methods such as waist circumference measurements, body fat percentage calculations, or progress photos. Focus on non-scale victories such as increased energy levels, improved strength and endurance, and enhanced mood and confidence.

In conclusion, understanding body composition is essential for assessing overall health, fitness, and well-being. By focusing on building a healthy body composition through strength training, cardiovascular exercise, a balanced diet, hydration, adequate sleep, stress management, and monitoring progress over time, you can optimize your body composition and support better health outcomes. Remember, every small step you take toward improving your body composition can have a positive impact on your quality of life and longevity.

CHAPTER 4:
MINDSET AND MOTIVATION

Welcome to a chapter dedicated to exploring the powerful role that mindset and motivation play in achieving weight loss and wellness goals. Your mindset—the way you perceive and interpret the world around you—and your level of motivation—the drive and determination to pursue your goals—are crucial factors that can either propel you forward or hold you back on your journey to better health. In this chapter, we'll delve into the importance of cultivating a positive mindset, strategies for staying motivated, and my personal experiences that have shaped my mindset and fueled my motivation along the way.

The Power of Mindset:

Your mindset shapes your beliefs, attitudes, and behaviours, ultimately influencing the choices you make and the actions you take. Adopting a positive mindset—one characterised by optimism, resilience, and self-belief—can empower you to overcome obstacles, bounce back from setbacks, and stay focused on your goals, even when faced with challenges.

Personal Experience: Growing up, I struggled with self-doubt and negative self-talk, which often hindered my ability to pursue my goals with confidence. However, through self-reflection, personal development, and surrounding myself with supportive individuals, I gradually shifted my mindset toward one of positivity and possibility. By reframing challenges as opportunities for growth and viewing setbacks as temporary setbacks rather than permanent failures, I was able to cultivate a mindset that propelled me forward on my journey to better health.

Strategies for Cultivating a Positive Mindset:

1. Practice Gratitude: Cultivate an attitude of gratitude by focusing on the positive aspects of your life and expressing appreciation for the blessings you have. Keep a gratitude journal, where you can write down three things you're thankful for each day, or simply take a few moments each morning or evening to reflect on the things that bring you joy and fulfilment.

2. Challenge Negative Thoughts: Become aware of negative thoughts and self-limiting beliefs that may be holding you back, and challenge them with positive affirmations and evidence to the contrary. Replace negative self-talk with words of encouragement and self-compassion, and remind

yourself of your strengths, accomplishments, and potential.

3. Set Realistic Goals: Break your larger goals into smaller, more manageable tasks and set realistic expectations for yourself. Enjoy your accomplishments as you go and resist the need to give up in the face of difficulties or setbacks. Remember that change takes time, and every small step you take toward your goals is a step in the right direction.

4. Surround Yourself with Positivity: Surround yourself with positive influences—whether it's supportive friends and family members, inspirational books and podcasts, or uplifting music and art—that uplift and motivate you. Limit exposure to negative influences, such as toxic relationships, pessimistic attitudes, and self-critical media, that drain your energy and dampen your spirits.

The Importance of Motivation:

Motivation is the driving force that propels you toward your goals and sustains your efforts over time. It's what keeps you focused, determined, and committed to taking action, even when faced with challenges or setbacks. Understanding what motivates you and how to maintain your motivation is essential for achieving long-term success.

Personal Experience: My journey to better health has been fueled by a deep-seated desire to live a vibrant, fulfilling life and to be the best version of myself that I can be. While there have been times when my motivation wavered, particularly in the face of obstacles or setbacks, I've always found ways to reignite my passion and recommit to my goals. Whether it's through visualising my desired outcomes, seeking support from loved ones, or reminding myself of the reasons why I started, I've learned to tap into my inner reserves of motivation and persevere in the face of adversity.

Strategies for Staying Motivated:

1. Define Your "Why": Clarify your reasons for wanting to achieve your goals and connect them to your values, passions, and aspirations. Ask yourself: What will achieving this goal mean to me? How will it improve my life and the lives of those around me? By anchoring your goals in a deeper sense of purpose and meaning, you'll be better equipped to stay motivated, even when faced with challenges.

2. Visualize Success: Create a mental image of what success looks and feels like for you, and visualize yourself achieving your goals with clarity and detail.

Use visualization techniques to imagine yourself overcoming obstacles, staying focused, and celebrating your achievements. By regularly visualizing your desired outcomes, you'll reinforce your motivation and strengthen your belief in your ability to succeed.

3. Break Goals into Actionable Steps: Break your goals down into smaller, more manageable tasks and create a plan of action for achieving them. Set specific, measurable, achievable, relevant, and time-bound (SMART) goals, and identify the actions you need to take to reach each milestone. By focusing on the process rather than the outcome, you'll maintain a sense of momentum and progress, which will fuel your motivation.

4. Find Your Tribe: Surround yourself with a supportive community of like-minded individuals who share your goals, values, and aspirations. Seek out accountability partners, mentors, coaches, or support groups who can offer encouragement, guidance, and accountability along your journey. By sharing your experiences, challenges, and successes with others, you'll feel more motivated, inspired, and connected.

5. Celebrate Progress: Acknowledge and celebrate your progress, no matter how small or insignificant it may seem. Take time to reflect on your

achievements, milestones, and breakthroughs, and reward yourself for your efforts. Whether it's treating yourself to a relaxing massage, enjoying a healthy meal, or simply patting yourself on the back, celebrating your progress will boost your morale and reinforce your motivation to keep going.

To sum up, motivation and mindset are strong factors that can either help us achieve our objectives or prevent us from reaching our greatest potential. By cultivating a positive mindset characterised by optimism, resilience, and self-belief, and by staying motivated through clarity of purpose, visualization, action planning, community support, and celebration of progress, we can overcome obstacles, stay focused, and achieve our goals. Remember, your mindset and motivation are within your control, so choose to cultivate habits and practices that uplift and empower you on your journey to better health and well-being.

Setting Realistic Goals

Welcome to a chapter dedicated to the art and science of setting realistic goals. Goal setting is a fundamental aspect of personal growth, achievement, and success. Whether you're embarking on a journey to improve your health, advance your career, or pursue personal passions, setting clear and achievable goals is essential for staying focused, motivated, and accountable. In this chapter, we'll explore the principles of effective goal setting, provide practical tips for setting realistic goals, and discuss how to stay on track and adjust your goals as needed along the way.

Understanding the Importance of Setting Realistic Goals:

Setting realistic goals is crucial for several reasons:

1. Clarity and Focus: Clear, well-defined goals provide direction and focus, helping you prioritize your time, energy, and resources toward what matters most to you. By knowing exactly what you want to achieve, you can align your actions and decisions with your desired outcomes, increasing your chances of success.

2. Motivation and Commitment: Realistic goals inspire motivation and commitment by giving you something tangible to work toward. When you set goals that are achievable and within reach, you're more likely to stay motivated and persevere in the face of obstacles or setbacks. Each small milestone you achieve reinforces your belief in your ability to succeed, fueling your determination to keep going.

3. Measurable Progress: Realistic goals are measurable, allowing you to track your progress and celebrate your achievements along the way. By breaking your larger goals into smaller, more manageable tasks and setting specific milestones, you can monitor your advancement and make adjustments as needed to stay on course.

4. Accountability and Evaluation: Setting realistic goals creates a framework for accountability and evaluation, holding you accountable for your actions and outcomes. By regularly reviewing your progress and assessing your performance against your goals, you can identify areas of strength and areas for improvement, enabling you to make informed decisions and adjustments to your approach.

Practical Tips for Setting Realistic Goals:

1. Define Your Objectives: Start by clarifying what you want to achieve and why it's important to you. Be specific and concrete in defining your objectives, and consider both short-term and long-term goals. Whether your goal is to lose weight, advance in your career, learn a new skill, or improve your relationships, clearly articulating your objectives will provide a solid foundation for goal setting.

2. Make Them SMART: Use the SMART criteria—Specific, Measurable, Achievable, Relevant, and Time-bound—to refine your goals and make them more actionable. Ensure that each goal is specific and clearly defined, measurable so that progress can be tracked, achievable given your current circumstances and resources, relevant to your overall objectives, and time-bound with a specific deadline or timeline for completion.

3. Break Them Down: Break your larger goals into smaller, more manageable tasks or sub-goals that you can tackle one step at a time. By breaking your goals down into smaller, bite-sized actions, you can make progress more manageable and reduce the feeling of overwhelm. Focus on what you can do today to move closer to your goals, rather than getting bogged down by the enormity of the task at hand.

4. Set Priorities: Prioritise your goals based on their importance and urgency, and focus your time and energy on the goals that will have the greatest impact on your life or well-being. Identify the goals that align most closely with your values, passions, and long-term aspirations, and allocate your resources accordingly. Remember that it's okay to say no to goals that aren't aligned with your priorities or that would stretch you too thin.

5. Consider Potential Obstacles: Anticipate potential obstacles or challenges that may arise along the way, and develop strategies for overcoming them. Whether it's lack of time, resources, or support, or fear of failure or rejection, identify potential barriers to goal achievement and brainstorm ways to address or mitigate them. By proactively planning for obstacles, you can increase your resilience and resourcefulness in the face of adversity.

6. Seek Support and Accountability: Share your goals with trusted friends, family members, mentors, or colleagues who can offer support, encouragement, and accountability. Having a support network of individuals who believe in your potential and are invested in your success can provide invaluable motivation and guidance along your journey. Consider joining a mastermind group, accountability partnership, or online community of like-minded individuals who share similar goals and aspirations.

7. Celebrate Your Progress: Celebrate your achievements and milestones along the way, no matter how small or insignificant they may seem. Take time to acknowledge your progress, reflect on your accomplishments, and reward yourself for your efforts. Whether it's treating yourself to a small indulgence, sharing your success with others, or simply taking a moment to pat yourself on the back, celebrating your progress reinforces your motivation and boosts your morale.

8. Stay Flexible and Adapt: Be open to adjusting your goals and plans as needed based on changing circumstances, feedback, or new information. Life is unpredictable, and it's essential to remain flexible and adaptable in the face of uncertainty. If you encounter unexpected challenges or opportunities, be willing to reassess your goals, revise your plans,

and pivot as necessary to stay on track and continue making progress toward your objectives.

In conclusion, setting realistic goals is essential for achieving success and fulfilment in all areas of life. By defining clear objectives, making them SMART, breaking them down into manageable tasks, setting priorities, considering potential obstacles, seeking support and accountability, celebrating progress, and staying flexible and adaptable,You have the ability to manifest your dreams and position yourself for success . Remember that goal setting is not a one-time event but an ongoing process of growth, learning, and self-discovery. Embrace the journey, stay focused on your goals, and enjoy the satisfaction of seeing your efforts pay off as you progress toward a brighter, more fulfilling future.

OVERCOMING MENTAL BLOCKS

Welcome to a chapter dedicated to exploring the common mental blocks that can hinder our progress and success, and practical strategies for overcoming them. Mental blocks are negative thought patterns, limiting beliefs, and self-imposed barriers that prevent us from reaching our full potential and achieving our goals. Whether it's self-doubt, fear of failure, perfectionism, or procrastination, these mental blocks can hold us back from pursuing our dreams and living a fulfilling life. In this chapter, we'll delve into the root causes of mental blocks, identify common types of mental blocks, and provide practical tips for overcoming them to unleash our true potential.

Understanding Mental Blocks:

Mental blocks can manifest in various forms and stem from a combination of internal and external factors. Some common types of mental blocks include:

1. Self-Doubt: Self-doubt is a pervasive mental block that undermines our confidence and belief in ourselves. It manifests as negative self-talk, feelings of inadequacy, and a lack of faith in our abilities. Self-doubt can stem from past failures, comparisons

to others, or negative feedback from others, and can paralyze us with fear and indecision.

2. Fear of Failure: Fear of failure is another common mental block that prevents us from taking risks and pursuing our goals. It manifests as a fear of making mistakes, facing rejection, or falling short of expectations. Fear of failure can stem from past experiences of disappointment or criticism, and can lead to procrastination, avoidance, and self-sabotage.

3. Perfectionism: Perfectionism is a mental block characterised by an unrelenting pursuit of flawlessness and an aversion to making mistakes or taking risks. It manifests as unrealistic standards, excessive self-criticism, and a fear of imperfection. Perfectionism can lead to procrastination, paralysis by analysis, and burnout, as we strive for unattainable ideals and judge ourselves harshly for falling short.

4. Procrastination: Procrastination is a mental block characterised by delaying or avoiding tasks or decisions that are necessary for achieving our goals. It manifests as distractions, excuses, and rationalisations for putting off important work. Procrastination can stem from fear, perfectionism, overwhelm, or lack of motivation, and can prevent us

from making progress and reaching our full
potential.

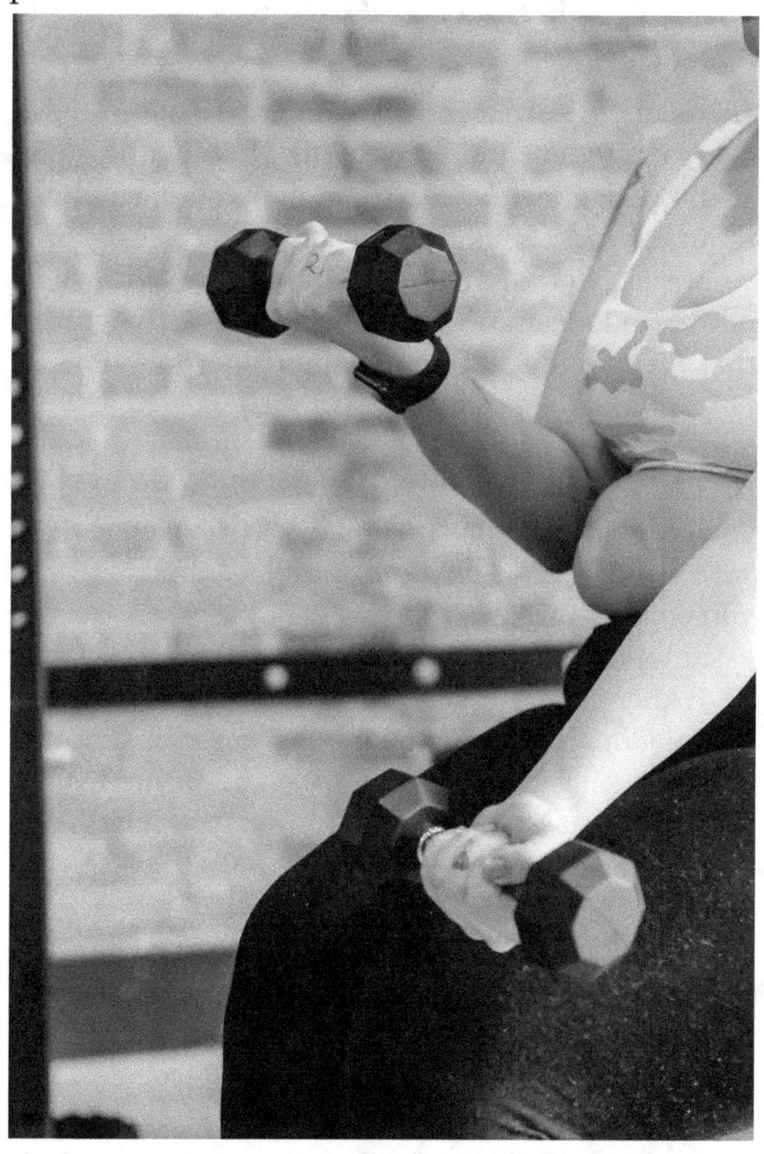

PRACTICAL TIPS FOR OVERCOMING MENTAL BLOCKS :

1. Identify Your Mental Blocks: The first step in overcoming mental blocks is to identify and acknowledge them. Take some time to reflect on the thoughts, beliefs, and behaviours that are holding you back from pursuing your goals. Write them down and examine them objectively, recognizing that they are not facts but rather interpretations or perceptions.

2. Challenge Your Negative Thoughts: Once you've identified your mental blocks, challenge them with evidence, logic, and rational thinking. Ask yourself: Is this thought or belief based on facts or assumptions? What proof do I have for it, or against it? Is there a more balanced or realistic perspective I could adopt? By challenging your negative thoughts and replacing them with more empowering beliefs, you can weaken their hold over you and open yourself up to new possibilities.

3. Cultivate Self-Compassion: Practise self-compassion by treating yourself with kindness, understanding, and acceptance, especially in moments of self-doubt or failure. Recognize that everyone experiences setbacks and struggles, and that your worth is not determined by your achievements or mistakes. Be gentle with yourself and offer yourself the same compassion and support that you would offer to a friend in a similar situation.

4. Set Realistic Expectations: Set realistic expectations for yourself and your goals, recognizing that progress is often incremental and that setbacks are a natural part of the learning process. Break your goals down into smaller, more manageable tasks, and focus on making steady progress rather than striving for perfection. Celebrate your achievements along the way, no matter how small, and adjust your goals as needed based on feedback and experience.

5. Take Action Despite Fear: Acknowledge your fears and insecurities, but don't let them dictate your actions or hold you back from pursuing your goals. Take small, manageable steps toward your goals, even if they feel uncomfortable or intimidating at first. Recall that bravery is the willingness to act in spite of fear, not the lack of it. By confronting your fears and pushing through your comfort zone, you'll build confidence and resilience over time.

6. Break Tasks into Smaller Steps: Break larger tasks or goals into smaller, more manageable steps, and focus on completing one step at a time. By breaking tasks down into bite-sized chunks, you'll reduce feelings of overwhelm and increase your sense of accomplishment as you make progress.

Celebrate each small victory along the way, and use momentum to propel you forward to the next step.

7. Practice Mindfulness and Relaxation Techniques: Incorporate mindfulness and relaxation techniques into your daily routine to reduce stress, quiet your mind, and increase self-awareness. Techniques such as deep breathing, meditation, yoga, and progressive muscle relaxation can help calm your nervous system, improve focus and concentration, and cultivate a sense of inner peace and balance. By practising mindfulness regularly, you'll become more adept at recognizing and managing your mental blocks as they arise.

8. Seek Support and Accountability: Reach out to friends, family members, mentors, or professional support networks for guidance, encouragement, and accountability. Share your goals and challenges with trusted individuals who can offer support, feedback, and perspective. Consider joining a support group, mastermind group, or online community of like-minded individuals who are also working to overcome mental blocks and pursue their goals. By surrounding yourself with a supportive network of people who believe in your potential and cheer you on, you'll feel more motivated, inspired, and empowered to overcome your mental blocks and achieve your goals.

In conclusion, overcoming mental blocks is essential for unlocking your full potential and achieving your goals. By identifying your mental blocks, challenging negative thoughts, cultivating self-compassion, setting realistic expectations, taking action despite fear, breaking tasks into smaller steps, practicing mindfulness and relaxation techniques, and seeking support and accountability, you can overcome the obstacles that stand in your way and create the life you desire. Remember that change takes time and effort, but with patience, perseverance, and the right strategies, you can break free from mental blocks and unleash your true potential.

FINDING INNER MOTIVATION

Welcome to a chapter dedicated to uncovering the power of inner motivation—the driving force that propels us toward our goals, sustains our efforts, and fuels our journey to success. Inner motivation, also known as intrinsic motivation, originates from within ourselves and is rooted in our personal values, passions, and aspirations. Unlike external motivators such as rewards or praise, inner motivation comes from a deep sense of purpose, meaning, and fulfilment. In this chapter, we'll explore the importance of finding inner motivation, share practical strategies for cultivating it, and delve into my personal experiences of discovering and harnessing my own inner motivation.

Understanding Inner Motivation:

Inner motivation is the fuel that ignites our desire to pursue our goals and aspirations, even in the face of challenges or setbacks. It is characterised by a sense of passion, purpose, and autonomy, and is driven by internal factors such as personal values, interests, and beliefs. Unlike external motivators such as money, fame, or approval from others, inner motivation comes from within ourselves and is deeply rooted in our sense of identity and self-expression.

Personal Experience: Throughout my life, I've encountered moments when external motivations—such as money, recognition, or social approval—failed to sustain my efforts or bring me lasting fulfilment. It wasn't until I discovered my inner motivation—the intrinsic desire to pursue goals that aligned with my values, passions, and purpose—that I truly felt inspired and empowered to take action. Whether it was pursuing a career in a field I was passionate about, committing to a fitness routine that nourished my body and soul, or embarking on a creative project that brought me joy and fulfilment, I found that tapping into my inner motivation was the key to unlocking my full potential and living a purpose-driven life.

Practical Strategies for Cultivating Inner Motivation:

1. Clarify Your Values and Priorities: Take some time to reflect on your core values, beliefs, and priorities in life. What matters most to you? What brings you a sense of fulfilment and meaning? By clarifying your values and priorities, you can align your goals and actions with what truly matters to you, giving you a sense of purpose and direction.

2. Connect with Your Passions: Identify activities, interests, and pursuits that ignite your passion and enthusiasm. What activities do you enjoy doing purely for the sake of doing them? What topics or subjects could you spend hours exploring without getting bored? By connecting with your passions and interests, you can tap into a deep reservoir of inner motivation that will drive you to pursue your goals with enthusiasm and commitment.

3. Set Meaningful Goals: Set goals that are meaningful, challenging, and aligned with your values and aspirations. What goals do you have for your life? What goals will bring you a sense of fulfilment and satisfaction? By setting meaningful goals that resonate with your values and aspirations, you'll feel a greater sense of purpose and motivation to pursue them with vigour and determination.

4. Find Your Why: Identify the underlying reasons why you want to achieve your goals. What is your driving force? What are you passionate about? By uncovering your "why"—the deeper purpose and meaning behind your goals—you'll tap into a powerful source of inner motivation that will keep you focused, resilient, and determined, even when faced with obstacles or setbacks.

5. Cultivate Intrinsic Rewards: Focus on the intrinsic rewards of pursuing your goals, such as personal growth, self-improvement, and mastery. What skills or abilities do you want to develop? What experiences do you want to have? By focusing on the intrinsic rewards of your efforts—such as the satisfaction of learning something new, the joy of creating something beautiful, or the sense of accomplishment from overcoming challenges—you'll fuel your inner motivation and sustain your efforts over the long term.

6. Practice Self-Compassion: Be kind and compassionate toward yourself as you pursue your goals and aspirations. Recognize that setbacks and failures are a natural part of the learning process, and treat yourself with the same kindness and understanding that you would offer to a friend facing similar challenges. By practising self-compassion, you'll cultivate a supportive inner dialogue that

encourages resilience, perseverance, and self-acceptance.

7. Foster Autonomy and Independence: Take ownership of your goals and actions, and cultivate a sense of autonomy and independence in pursuing them. What steps can you take to take control of your life and make decisions that align with your values and aspirations? By fostering autonomy and independence, you'll feel a greater sense of empowerment and agency in shaping your destiny, fueling your inner motivation to pursue your goals with confidence and determination.

8. Seek Inspiration and Support: Surround yourself with people, resources, and environments that inspire and support your goals and aspirations. Seek out mentors, role models, and like-minded individuals who share your values and passions, and draw inspiration from their experiences and achievements. By surrounding yourself with a supportive community of individuals who believe in your potential and cheer you on, you'll feel encouraged, motivated, and empowered to pursue your goals with enthusiasm and determination.

In conclusion, finding inner motivation is essential for unleashing your full potential and living a purpose-driven life. By clarifying your values and priorities, connecting with your passions, setting meaningful goals, finding your why, cultivating intrinsic rewards, practicing self-compassion, fostering autonomy and independence, and seeking inspiration and support, you can tap into a deep reservoir of inner motivation that will propel you toward your goals with passion, purpose, and perseverance. Remember that inner motivation is within your control, and by nurturing it with care and intention, you can achieve anything you set your mind to and create a life that is rich, meaningful, and fulfilling.

CHAPTER 5:
NUTRITION ESSENTIALS

Welcome to a chapter dedicated to understanding the fundamental principles of nutrition and how they relate to your health and well-being. Nutrition plays a crucial role in fueling your body, supporting your overall health, and optimizing your performance in various aspects of life. In this chapter, we'll explore the essentials of nutrition, providing practical tips for making informed food choices, building balanced meals, and cultivating healthy eating habits that promote vitality and longevity.

Understanding Macronutrients:

Macronutrients are the three main components of food that provide energy and essential nutrients for your body: carbohydrates, proteins, and fats.

1. Carbohydrates: Carbohydrates are your body's primary source of energy, providing fuel for your brain, muscles, and other organs. They come in two main forms: simple carbohydrates, found in foods like fruits, vegetables, and sweets, and complex carbohydrates, found in foods like whole grains, legumes, and starchy vegetables. Aim to include a variety of carbohydrates in your diet, focusing on

whole, unprocessed sources that provide fiber, vitamins, and minerals.

2. Proteins: Proteins are essential for building and repairing tissues, synthesizing hormones and enzymes, and supporting immune function. Amino acids, sometimes known as the "building blocks" of protein, are what make them up. Include a variety of protein sources in your diet, such as lean meats, poultry, fish, eggs, dairy products, legumes, nuts, and seeds, to ensure you're getting all the essential amino acids your body needs.

3. Fats: Fats are essential for energy production, nutrient absorption, hormone regulation, and cell membrane structure. They come in several forms, including saturated fats, unsaturated fats, and trans fats. Focus on including healthy fats in your diet, such as monounsaturated and polyunsaturated fats found in foods like avocados, olive oil, nuts, seeds, and fatty fish, while limiting your consumption of processed meals, fried foods, and fatty meats that are high in saturated and trans fats.

Balancing Your Plate:

Building balanced meals is key to meeting your nutritional needs and maintaining optimal health. Aim to include a variety of nutrient-dense foods from all food groups in each meal, focusing on the following components:

1. Vegetables: Fill half of your plate with non-starchy vegetables, such as leafy greens, broccoli, carrots, bell peppers, and tomatoes. These foods are rich in vitamins, minerals, fiber, and antioxidants, and are low in calories, making them an essential component of a balanced diet.

2. Protein: Include a palm-sized portion of lean protein with each meal, such as chicken, turkey, fish, tofu, tempeh, beans, lentils, or eggs. Protein helps to satisfy hunger, stabilize blood sugar levels, and support muscle growth and repair.

3. Carbohydrates: Add a fist-sized portion of carbohydrates to your plate, choosing whole, unprocessed sources like brown rice, quinoa, sweet potatoes, whole grain bread, or legumes. These foods provide sustained energy and fiber, helping to keep you feeling full and satisfied.

4. Healthy Fats: Incorporate a thumb-sized portion of healthy fats into your meals, such as avocado,

olive oil, nuts, seeds, or fatty fish like salmon or trout. Healthy fats provide essential fatty acids and fat-soluble vitamins, as well as flavor and satiety.

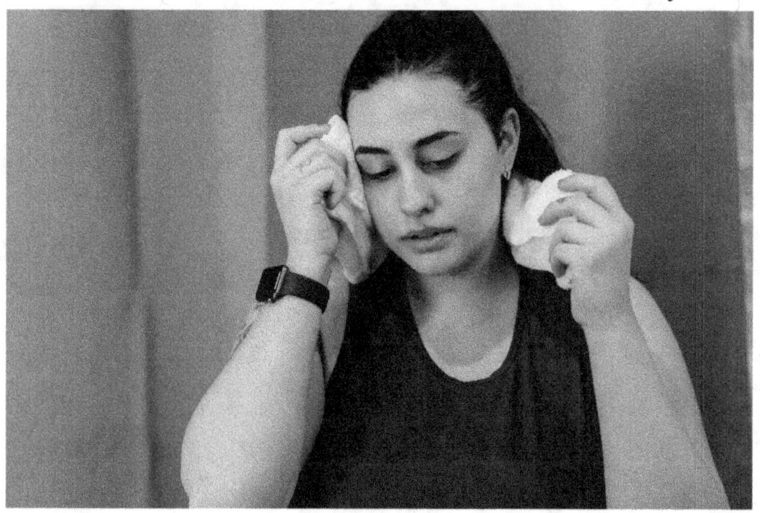

Practical Tips for Healthy Eating:

1. Focus on Whole Foods: Choose whole, unprocessed foods whenever possible, such as fruits, vegetables, whole grains, lean proteins, and healthy fats. These foods are rich in nutrients and fiber and are free from added sugars, refined grains, and artificial additives.

2. Read Food Labels: When purchasing packaged foods, read the nutrition labels carefully to understand the ingredients and nutritional content. Pay attention to serving sizes, calorie counts, and the amounts of macronutrients, vitamins, and minerals per serving.

3. Stay Hydrated: Drink plenty of water throughout the day to stay hydrated and support optimal bodily functions. Aim for at least 8-10 glasses of water per day, and more if you're physically active or in hot weather.

4. Practice Portion Control: Be mindful of portion sizes and avoid overeating by listening to your body's hunger and fullness cues. Reduce the size of your dishes, plates, and utensils to help you eat less and avoid overindulging.

5. Cook at Home: Prepare meals at home whenever possible, using fresh, whole ingredients and cooking

methods like baking, grilling, steaming, or sautéing. Cooking at home allows you to control the ingredients and cooking methods, making it easier to make healthier choices.

6. Limit Processed Foods: Minimize your intake of processed and ultra-processed foods like sugary snacks, sweetened beverages, fried foods, and packaged meals, which are often high in added sugars, unhealthy fats, and sodium.

7. Practice Mindful Eating: Slow down and savor each bite of your meals, paying attention to the flavors, textures, and sensations of eating. Eat without distractions, such as watching TV or scrolling on your phone, to fully enjoy your food and tune into your body's hunger and fullness signals.

8. Seek Professional Guidance: If you have specific dietary needs or health concerns, consider seeking guidance from a registered dietitian or nutritionist who can provide personalized recommendations and support.

In conclusion, nutrition is a cornerstone of health and well-being, providing the essential nutrients your body needs to function optimally and thrive. By understanding the basics of nutrition, building balanced meals, and adopting healthy eating habits, you can nourish your body, support your health goals, and enjoy a vibrant, energetic life. Remember to focus on whole, unprocessed foods, practice portion control, stay hydrated, and listen to your body's hunger and fullness cues to fuel your body with the nutrients it needs to thrive.

THE IMPORTANCE OF A BALANCED DIET

Eating is not just about filling our stomachs; it's about nourishing our bodies. A balanced diet is like the conductor of an orchestra, ensuring that every part of our body functions harmoniously. In this chapter, we'll explore why a balanced diet is crucial for overall health and well-being. We'll also provide practical tips to help you achieve and maintain a balanced diet in your daily life.

Why is a Balanced Diet Important?

Think of your body as a machine that needs different fuels to run smoothly. Just as a car needs the right mix of gas, oil, and coolant, our bodies require a variety of nutrients to function properly. Here's why a balanced diet matters:

1. Energy and Vitality: Food is our body's fuel. A balanced diet provides the energy needed for everyday activities, whether it's walking, working, or playing. Carbohydrates, fats, and proteins are the primary sources of energy, and a balanced diet ensures we get them in the right proportions to maintain vitality throughout the day.

2. Nutrient Supply: Our bodies need various vitamins and minerals to grow, repair tissues, and regulate bodily functions. A balanced diet rich in fruits, vegetables, whole grains, lean proteins, and healthy fats ensures we get the essential nutrients necessary for optimal health and well-being.

3. Weight Management: Maintaining a healthy weight is essential for reducing the risk of chronic diseases like diabetes, heart disease, and certain cancers. A balanced diet, combined with regular physical activity, helps us achieve and maintain a healthy weight by providing the right balance of nutrients without excess calories.

4. Brain Function: Our brains need proper nutrition to stay sharp and focused. Omega-3 fatty acids, found in foods like fish and nuts, are crucial for brain health, while antioxidants from fruits and vegetables help protect brain cells from damage.

5. Digestive Health: A balanced diet rich in fiber promotes a healthy digestive system by preventing constipation and supporting the growth of beneficial gut bacteria. This, in turn, boosts immunity and reduces the risk of digestive disorders.

6. Heart Health: High cholesterol levels and high blood pressure are significant risk factors for heart disease. A balanced diet low in saturated fats and

sodium, and high in fruits, vegetables, and whole grains, can help lower these risk factors and protect your heart.

7. Mood and Mental Well-being: What we eat can also affect our mood and mental health. Certain nutrients, such as serotonin precursors found in foods like turkey and bananas, can help regulate mood and promote feelings of happiness and relaxation.

Practical Tips for Achieving a Balanced Diet

Now that we know how important a balanced diet is, let's look at some useful advice to help you get one:

1. Eat a Variety of Foods: Aim to include foods from all food groups in your meals. Each food group provides different nutrients, so by eating a variety of foods, you ensure you get a wide range of essential nutrients.

2. Portion Control: To prevent overindulging, be mindful of portion sizes. Minimize portion sizes and avoid mindless eating by using smaller bowls, plates, and utensils.

3. Focus on Whole Foods: Choose whole, minimally processed foods over highly processed ones whenever possible. Whole foods are richer in nutrients and usually lower in added sugars, sodium, and unhealthy fats.

4. Plan Ahead: Take time to plan your meals and snacks for the week ahead. Planning ahead can help you make healthier choices and avoid impulsive, unhealthy food choices.

5. Remain Hydrated: To stay hydrated, sip lots of water throughout the day. Sometimes, feelings of hunger are actually signs of dehydration, so reach for water first when you feel hungry between meals.

6. Pay Attention to Your Body: Observe the signals your body sends when it is hungry or full. Rather than eating because you're bored or out of habit, eat when you're hungry and quit when you're satisfied.

7. Limit Added Sugars and Saturated Fats: Be mindful of your intake of added sugars and saturated fats, as these can contribute to weight gain and increase the risk of chronic diseases. Opt for healthier alternatives like natural sweeteners and unsaturated fats whenever possible.

8. Be Flexible: Remember that balance is key, and it's okay to indulge in your favorite treats

occasionally. The goal is not perfection but rather consistency and moderation in your overall eating habits.

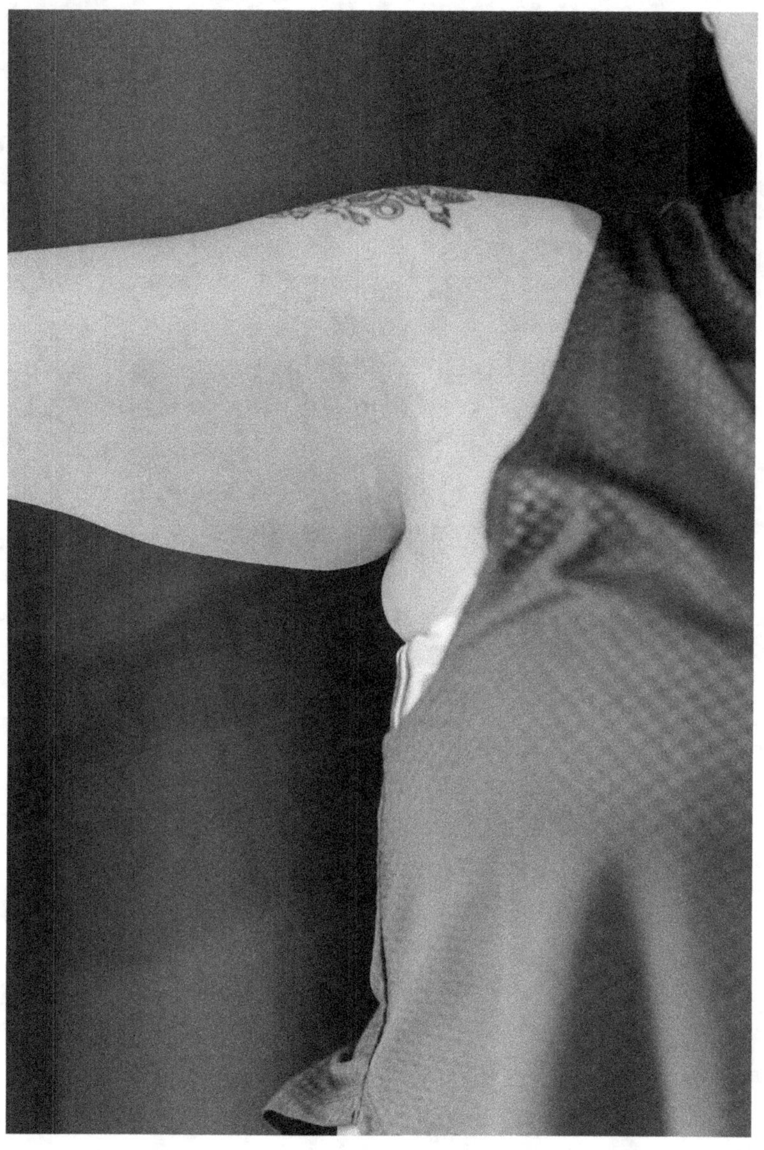

By incorporating these practical tips into your daily life, you can achieve a balanced diet that supports your overall health and well-being. Remember, small changes can lead to significant improvements in your health over time. So, take it one step at a time, and enjoy the journey to a healthier you!

Nutrient Requirements for Women Over 45

Women's bodies change as they get older, which may have an impact on what they need to eat. Maintaining a healthy diet becomes even more critical to support overall health and well-being. In this chapter, we'll discuss the specific nutrient requirements for women over 45 and provide practical tips to help meet these needs.

Nutrient Requirements for Women Over 45

As women enter their midlife and beyond, several factors can influence their nutrient requirements. These include hormonal changes, changes in metabolism, and the risk of certain health conditions. Here are some key nutrients that women over 45 should pay attention to:

1. Calcium: Calcium is essential for maintaining strong bones and preventing osteoporosis, a condition characterized by bone loss and increased risk of fractures. Women over 45 need around 1,200

milligrams of calcium per day, which can be obtained from dairy products, leafy greens, tofu, and fortified foods.

2. Vitamin D: Vitamin D is crucial for calcium absorption and bone health. As women age, their ability to produce vitamin D from sunlight decreases, making it important to get an adequate intake from food sources such as fatty fish, egg yolks, fortified dairy products, and supplements if necessary. The recommended daily intake for vitamin D is 600-800 IU for women over 45.

3. Fiber: Fiber is essential for maintaining digestive health and preventing constipation, which becomes more common with age. Women over 45 should aim for 21-25 grams of fiber per day from sources such as fruits, vegetables, whole grains, nuts, and seeds.

4. Iron: Iron requirements decrease after menopause for women due to the cessation of menstruation. However, it's still essential to ensure an adequate intake to prevent iron deficiency anaemia. Good sources of iron include lean meats, poultry, fish, beans, lentils, tofu, fortified cereals, and dark leafy greens.

5. Omega-3 Fatty Acids: Omega-3 fatty acids have anti-inflammatory properties and are beneficial for heart health, cognitive function, and joint health.

Women over 45 can include sources of omega-3s such as fatty fish (salmon, mackerel, sardines), flaxseeds, chia seeds, walnuts, and soybeans in their diet.

6. B Vitamins: B vitamins play a crucial role in energy metabolism, nerve function, and red blood cell production. As women age, their ability to absorb vitamin B12 from food may decrease, so it's important to include sources such as lean meats, fish, poultry, eggs, dairy products, and fortified foods. Other B vitamins, including B6, B9 (folate), and B2 (riboflavin), can be obtained from a varied diet that includes whole grains, fruits, vegetables, and legumes.

7. Magnesium: Magnesium is involved in hundreds of biochemical reactions in the body, including muscle and nerve function, blood sugar regulation, and bone health. Women over 45 should aim for around 320 milligrams of magnesium per day from sources such as nuts, seeds, whole grains, leafy greens, and legumes.

PRACTICAL TIPS FOR MEETING NUTRIENT REQUIREMENTS

Now that we've discussed the specific nutrient requirements for women over 45, let's explore some practical tips to help meet these needs:

1. Eat a Balanced Diet: Focus on consuming a variety of nutrient-dense foods from all food groups, including fruits, vegetables, whole grains, lean proteins, and healthy fats.

2. Include Calcium-Rich Foods: Incorporate dairy products, leafy greens, tofu, almonds, and calcium-fortified foods into your diet to ensure an adequate intake of calcium for bone health.

3. Get Plenty of Vitamin D: Spend time outdoors in sunlight when possible and include vitamin D-rich foods like fatty fish, egg yolks, fortified dairy products, and supplements as needed to maintain optimal vitamin D levels.

4. Prioritize Fiber: Choose whole grains, fruits, vegetables, nuts, and seeds to increase your fiber intake and support digestive health.

5. Vary Your Protein Sources: Include a variety of protein sources in your diet, such as lean meats,

poultry, fish, beans, lentils, tofu, and dairy products, to ensure adequate intake of essential amino acids.

6. Incorporate Omega-3s: Consume fatty fish, flaxseeds, chia seeds, walnuts, and soybeans regularly to obtain omega-3 fatty acids for heart and brain health.

7. Consider Supplements: Consult with a healthcare professional to determine if you need supplements to address specific nutrient deficiencies or to support overall health and well-being.

8. Stay Hydrated: Drink plenty of water throughout the day to stay hydrated and support overall health.

9. Limit Processed Foods and Added Sugars: Minimize consumption of processed foods, sugary snacks, and beverages, as they often lack essential nutrients and can contribute to health issues such as weight gain and inflammation.

By following these practical tips and prioritizing nutrient-rich foods, women over 45 can ensure they meet their specific nutrient requirements and support their overall health and well-being as they age. Remember to listen to your body's cues, stay active, and prioritize self-care to maintain optimal health in the years to come.

EMBRACING HEALTHY EATING HABITS

Eating is not merely about satisfying hunger; it's a fundamental aspect of self-care and well-being. Healthy eating habits play a pivotal role in shaping our physical health, mental clarity, and overall quality of life. In this chapter, we'll delve into the essence of healthy eating habits, exploring their significance and sharing personal experiences that highlight their transformative power.

Understanding Healthy Eating Habits

Eating properly does not mean following rigid dietary guidelines or denying yourself of your favorite foods. Instead, it's about making mindful choices that nourish your body and support your health goals. It's about finding a balance that works for you, where nutritious foods form the foundation of your diet while still allowing room for occasional treats.

My Journey Towards Healthy Eating

Growing up, my relationship with food was a rollercoaster of indulgence and guilt. I often found myself reaching for convenient, processed snacks to satisfy cravings or provide comfort during stressful times. However, as I became more aware of the impact of my food choices on my well-being, I embarked on a journey towards adopting healthier eating habits.

One of the most significant shifts in my approach to food was prioritising whole, unprocessed foods over packaged convenience items. I started incorporating more fruits, vegetables, whole grains, and lean proteins into my meals, gradually crowding out the less nutritious options. Not only did this change improve my physical health, but it also enhanced my energy levels and mental clarity.

Key Principles of Healthy Eating

1. Eat a Rainbow: Aim to include a variety of colorful fruits and vegetables in your meals to ensure you're getting a wide range of vitamins, minerals, and antioxidants. Think of each color as a different nutrient powerhouse, from the vibrant red of tomatoes to the deep green of kale.

2. Make Whole Foods Your Top Priority: Give foods that are closest to nature's original state priority. Whole grains, legumes, nuts, seeds, and fresh produce should form the basis of your diet, providing essential nutrients and fiber to support digestion and overall health.

3. Mindful Eating: Slow down and savor each bite, paying attention to hunger and fullness cues. Mindful eating helps prevent overeating and promotes a deeper connection with the food we consume, fostering gratitude and appreciation for nourishing our bodies.

4. Stay Hydrated: Water is essential for proper hydration, digestion, and overall health. Make it a habit to drink water throughout the day, and consider flavoring it with fresh herbs, fruit slices, or cucumber for added enjoyment.

5. Plan Ahead: Set yourself up for success by planning your meals and snacks in advance. This can help prevent impulsive, unhealthy food choices and ensure you have nutritious options readily available when hunger strikes.

6. Practice Moderation: Healthy eating isn't about perfection; it's about balance. Allow yourself to enjoy your favorite treats in moderation, savoring each indulgence without guilt. Remember that it's the overall pattern of your eating habits that matters most.

THE TRANSFORMATIVE POWER OF HEALTHY EATING

As I embraced healthier eating habits, I noticed profound changes in both my physical and emotional well-being. I felt more energized, resilient, and focused, able to tackle life's challenges with greater ease. My relationship with food shifted from one of restriction and guilt to one of nourishment and joy, enhancing not only my health but also my overall quality of life.

Conclusion

Healthy eating habits are a cornerstone of holistic well-being, empowering us to thrive physically, mentally, and emotionally. By prioritizing whole, nutritious foods, practicing mindfulness, and embracing balance, we can cultivate a lifelong relationship with food that nourishes and sustains us on our journey towards optimal health and vitality. Together, let's set out on this trip, one healthful mouthful at a time.

CHAPTER 6:

EXERCISE FOR WOMEN OVER 45

Exercise is not just about looking good; it's about feeling great and staying healthy as we age. For women over 45, staying active becomes even more important to maintain strength, flexibility, and overall well-being. In this chapter, we'll discuss the benefits of exercise for women in this age group and provide practical tips to help incorporate physical activity into their daily lives.

Benefits of Exercise for Women Over 45

1. Bone Health: As women age, they become more susceptible to osteoporosis, a condition characterised by weak and brittle bones. Weight-bearing exercises, such as walking, jogging, dancing, and strength training, help maintain bone density and reduce the risk of fractures.

2. Muscle Strength and Tone: Loss of muscle mass and strength is a natural part of aging, but regular exercise can help counteract this decline. Strength training exercises, using resistance bands, free weights, or bodyweight exercises, help build and maintain muscle strength and tone.

3. Heart Health: Heart disease is a leading cause of death among women, especially as they get older. Engaging in aerobic exercises, such as brisk walking, cycling, swimming, or dancing, helps improve cardiovascular health by strengthening the heart and improving circulation.

4. Weight Management: Metabolism tends to slow down with age, making it easier to gain weight. Regular exercise helps boost metabolism, burn calories, and maintain a healthy weight, reducing the risk of obesity and related health issues like diabetes and high blood pressure.

5. Joint Health and Flexibility: Joint stiffness and reduced flexibility are common complaints as women age. Stretching exercises, yoga, and tai chi can help improve joint mobility, reduce stiffness, and enhance overall flexibility, making daily activities easier and more comfortable.

6. Mental Well-being: Exercise is not only beneficial for the body but also for the mind. Physical activity releases endorphins, chemicals in the brain that promote feelings of happiness and reduce stress and anxiety. Regular exercise can also improve sleep quality and boost self-esteem and confidence.

Practical Tips for Exercise

1. Start Slowly: If you're new to exercise or haven't been active for a while, start slowly and gradually increase the intensity and duration of your workouts. Pay attention to your body's needs and refrain from overexerting oneself, particularly in the beginning.

2. Find Activities You Enjoy: Exercise doesn't have to be boring or tedious. Choose activities that you enjoy and look forward to, whether it's walking in nature, dancing to your favorite music, or practicing yoga in the comfort of your home.

3. Mix It Up: Incorporate a variety of exercises into your routine to keep things interesting and target different muscle groups. Include aerobic activities for cardiovascular health, strength training for muscle strength, and flexibility exercises for joint mobility.

4. Set Realistic Goals: Set achievable goals based on your current fitness level and lifestyle. Whether it's walking a certain distance, lifting a certain weight, or mastering a new yoga pose, setting realistic goals can help keep you motivated and focused.

5. Stay Consistent: Consistency is key to seeing results from your exercise routine. In addition to at least 150 minutes of moderate-intensity aerobic

activity or 75 minutes of vigorous-intensity activity per week, aim for two or more days of muscle-strengthening activities.

6. Pay Attention to Your Body: Observe your body's reaction to exercise and recovery. If you experience pain or discomfort, stop and rest or modify your workout as needed. It's essential to prioritise safety and avoid overdoing it to prevent injury.

7. Include Balance and Stability Exercises: As we age, maintaining balance and stability becomes increasingly important to prevent falls and injuries. Include exercises that challenge balance, such as standing on one leg or using balance boards or stability balls.

8. Stay Hydrated and Fuel Your Body: Drink plenty of water before, during, and after exercise to stay hydrated, and fuel your body with nutritious foods to support energy levels and recovery.

Recall that there is always time to begin enjoying the advantages of physical activity. By incorporating regular physical activity into your daily routine and following these practical tips, women over 45 can improve their health, vitality, and overall quality of life. So, lace up those sneakers, put on your favorite workout gear, and get moving towards a healthier, happier you!

TYPES OF EXERCISE FOR WEIGHT LOSS

Losing weight is a common goal for many people, and exercise plays a crucial role in achieving it. However, with so many exercise options available, it can be overwhelming to know where to start. In this chapter, we'll explore various types of exercise that are effective for weight loss and provide practical tips to help you incorporate them into your routine.

1. Aerobic Exercise

Aerobic exercise, also known as cardio, is one of the most effective forms of exercise for burning calories and promoting weight loss. It involves repetitive, rhythmic movements that increase your heart rate and breathing rate. Some popular aerobic exercises include:

- Walking: Walking is a low-impact exercise that can be done almost anywhere and requires no special equipment. Aim for brisk walking sessions lasting at least 30 minutes to an hour to burn calories and boost metabolism.

- Running or Jogging: Running or jogging is a high-impact aerobic exercise that can torch calories and build cardiovascular endurance. Start with short intervals of running or jogging, gradually increasing the duration and intensity as your fitness improves.

- Cycling: Cycling, whether outdoors or on a stationary bike, is a great way to burn calories and improve cardiovascular health. Try cycling at a moderate to vigorous intensity for optimal weight loss benefits.

- Swimming: Swimming is a full-body workout that engages multiple muscle groups while providing a low-impact cardiovascular workout. It's an excellent option for those with joint pain or mobility issues.

- Dancing: Dancing is a fun and enjoyable way to get your heart pumping and burn calories. Whether it's salsa, Zumba, or hip-hop, dancing can be a great way to improve fitness and lose weight while having a blast.

Practical Tips for Aerobic Exercise for Weight Loss:

- Choose Activities You Enjoy: Find aerobic activities that you genuinely enjoy to make exercise more enjoyable and sustainable in the long run.

- Gradually Increase Intensity: Start with a comfortable intensity and gradually increase the intensity and duration of your aerobic workouts as your fitness improves.

- Mix It Up: Incorporate a variety of aerobic exercises into your routine to prevent boredom and keep your body challenged.

2. Strength Training

Strength training, also known as resistance training, is essential for building lean muscle mass and boosting metabolism. While it may not burn as many calories during the workout as aerobic exercise, it helps increase muscle mass, which in turn increases calorie burn at rest. Some effective strength training exercises include:

- Bodyweight Exercises: Exercises such as squats, lunges, push-ups, and planks use your body weight as resistance and can be done anywhere, with no equipment required.

- Weightlifting: Using dumbbells, barbells, kettlebells, or resistance bands, weightlifting exercises target specific muscle groups to build strength and increase muscle mass.

- Resistance Machines: Gym machines like leg press, chest press, and lat pulldown provide guided resistance training for various muscle groups and are suitable for beginners and advanced exercisers alike.

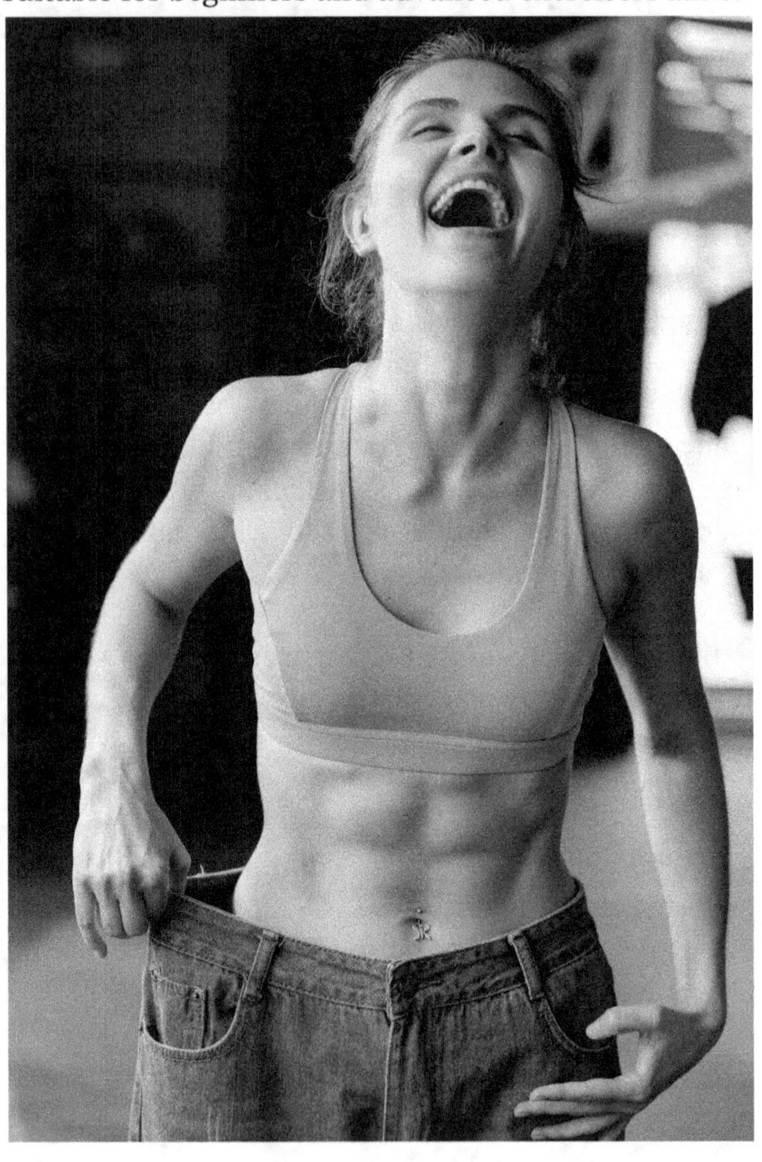

Practical Tips for Strength Training for Weight Loss:

- Focus on Compound Movements: Compound exercises that target multiple muscle groups, such as squats, deadlifts, and bench presses, are highly effective for building strength and burning calories.

- Progressively Overload: Gradually increase the resistance or repetitions of your strength training exercises over time to continue challenging your muscles and promoting muscle growth.

- Include Rest Days: Allow your muscles time to recover and repair by incorporating rest days into your strength training routine. Aim for at least 48 hours of rest between sessions targeting the same muscle groups.

3. High-Intensity Interval Training (HIIT)

High-Intensity Interval Training (HIIT) involves alternating short bursts of intense exercise with brief periods of rest or lower-intensity exercise. HIIT exercises are well-known for their effectiveness in increasing cardiovascular fitness and burning calories. Some examples of HIIT exercises include:

- Sprinting Intervals: Alternate between short sprints and periods of walking or jogging to elevate your heart rate and maximize calorie burn.

- Tabata Training: Complete exercises at maximum effort for 20 seconds, then take a 10-second break. Repeat this sequence numerous times

- Circuit Training: Combine strength training exercises with cardio intervals in a circuit format, moving quickly from one exercise to the next with minimal rest.

Practical Tips for HIIT for Weight Loss:

- Start Slowly: If you're not familiar with HIIT, begin with shorter intervals and work your way up to longer and more intense ones as your fitness level increases.

- Listen to Your Body: Pay attention to how your body responds to HIIT workouts and adjust the intensity or duration as needed to avoid overexertion and injury.

- Include Recovery Periods: Allow adequate time for recovery between HIIT sessions to prevent burnout and promote muscle repair and growth.

4. Flexibility and Mobility Exercises

While flexibility and mobility exercises may not directly contribute to calorie burn like aerobic or strength training, they play a crucial role in overall fitness and weight loss success. Improving flexibility and mobility can enhance exercise performance, reduce the risk of injury, and support recovery. Exercises for improving flexibility and mobility include the following:

- Yoga: Yoga combines stretching, strength, and relaxation techniques to improve flexibility, balance, and mental well-being.

- Pilates: Using deliberate movements and breathing techniques, Pilates emphasizes body awareness, flexibility, and core strength.

- Foam Rolling: Foam rolling helps release muscle tension and improve flexibility by applying pressure to tight or sore muscles using a foam roller.

Practical Tips for Flexibility and Mobility Exercises:

- Incorporate into Your Routine: Include flexibility and mobility exercises as part of your warm-up or cool-down routine before and after aerobic or strength training workouts.

- Focus on Proper Form: Pay attention to proper alignment and technique during flexibility exercises to maximize their effectiveness and reduce the risk of injury.

- Be Consistent: Consistency is key to seeing improvements in flexibility and mobility. Aim to practice flexibility exercises regularly to maintain and gradually improve your range of motion.

In conclusion, there are various types of exercise that can contribute to weight loss and overall health. By incorporating a combination of aerobic exercise, strength training, HIIT, and flexibility exercises into your routine, you can optimize calorie burn, build muscle mass, improve cardiovascular health, and enhance flexibility and mobility. Remember to start gradually, listen to your body, and choose activities that you enjoy to make exercise a sustainable and enjoyable part of your lifestyle.

STRENGTH TRAINING FOR OLDER WOMEN

Strength training is a powerful tool for improving overall health and well-being, especially as we age. Contrary to common misconceptions, strength training is not just for bodybuilders or athletes—it's for everyone, including older women. In this chapter, we'll discuss the benefits of strength training for older women and provide practical tips to help them incorporate it into their lives.

Benefits of Strength Training for Older Women

Strength training offers a multitude of benefits that are particularly valuable for older women:

1. Increased Muscle Mass: As we age, we naturally lose muscle mass and strength. Strength training helps counteract this decline by stimulating muscle growth and improving muscle tone, making everyday tasks easier and reducing the risk of falls and injuries.

2. Improved Bone Health: Strength training is not only beneficial for muscles but also for bones. By applying stress to the bones through resistance exercises, strength training helps maintain or even

increase bone density, reducing the risk of osteoporosis and fractures.

3. Enhanced Metabolism: Building and maintaining lean muscle mass through strength training can boost metabolism, helping older women burn more calories at rest and support weight management.

4. Better Joint Health: Strength training exercises that target the muscles around the joints can help improve joint stability and function, reducing pain and stiffness associated with conditions like arthritis.

5. Improved Mood and Mental Health: Strength training releases endorphins, chemicals in the brain that promote feelings of happiness and reduce stress and anxiety. Regular strength training can also boost self-esteem and confidence, leading to better overall mental well-being.

Practical Tips for Strength Training for Older Women

1. Start Slowly and Progress Gradually: If you're new to strength training or have been inactive for a while, start with light weights or resistance bands and focus on mastering proper form before increasing the intensity. Gradually increase the weight or resistance

as you become stronger and more comfortable with the exercises.

2. Choose the Right Exercises: Focus on compound exercises that target multiple muscle groups, such as squats, lunges, push-ups, rows, and overhead presses. These exercises are efficient and effective for building strength and functional fitness.

3. Use Proper Form: Proper form is essential for maximizing the effectiveness of strength training exercises and reducing the risk of injury. Take the time to learn the correct technique for each exercise, and don't hesitate to ask for guidance from a qualified fitness professional if needed.

4. Incorporate Balance and Stability Exercises: As we age, maintaining balance and stability becomes increasingly important for preventing falls and injuries. Include balance and stability exercises, such as single-leg stands, heel-to-toe walks, and stability ball exercises, in your strength training routine to improve proprioception and coordination.

5. Listen to Your Body: Pay attention to how your body responds to strength training exercises and adjust the intensity or volume accordingly. It's normal to experience some muscle soreness, but if you feel pain or discomfort beyond typical muscle

fatigue, it's important to back off and rest or modify the exercise.

6. Prioritise Recovery: Allow your muscles time to recover and repair between strength training sessions. Aim for at least 48 hours of rest between workouts targeting the same muscle groups to prevent overtraining and promote muscle growth.

7. Stay Consistent: Consistency is key to seeing results from strength training. Aim for at least two to three strength training sessions per week, with a day of rest in between each session, to build and maintain strength effectively.

8. Warm Up and Cool Down: Always start your strength training sessions with a proper warm-up to prepare your muscles and joints for exercise, and finish with a cool-down to help reduce muscle soreness and promote recovery. Warm up with dynamic stretches and mobility exercises, and cool down with static stretches.

9. Use Proper Equipment: Invest in comfortable, supportive workout attire and proper footwear to ensure safety and comfort during strength training sessions. If using free weights or resistance bands, choose appropriate resistance levels that challenge you without compromising form.

10. Listen to Your Body: Pay attention to any signs of discomfort or pain during exercise, and modify or stop any movements that cause pain. It's essential to prioritise safety and avoid overexertion to prevent injury.

By following these practical tips and incorporating strength training into your routine, older women can reap the numerous benefits of improved strength, bone health, metabolism, and overall well-being. Remember that it's never too late to start strength training, and consistency is key to seeing results over time. So, lace up those sneakers, grab some weights or resistance bands, and start building a stronger, healthier you today!

CARDIOVASCULAR EXERCISE AND ITS BENEFITS

Cardiovascular exercise, often referred to simply as cardio, is a cornerstone of physical fitness. It involves activities that elevate your heart rate and increase blood circulation, providing a wide array of health benefits. In this chapter, we'll explore the importance of cardiovascular exercise and discuss its numerous benefits. Additionally, we'll provide practical tips to help you incorporate cardio into your routine and make the most of its advantages.

Understanding Cardiovascular Exercise

Cardiovascular exercise encompasses any activity that gets your heart pumping and increases your breathing rate. It includes a variety of exercises, from brisk walking and jogging to cycling, swimming, dancing, and aerobics. The primary goal of cardiovascular exercise is to improve the health of your heart and circulatory system, enhancing overall fitness and well-being.

Benefits of Cardiovascular Exercise

1. Improved Heart Health: Cardiovascular exercise strengthens the heart muscle, enabling it to pump blood more efficiently throughout the body. Over

time, regular cardio can lower blood pressure, reduce the risk of heart disease, and improve overall cardiovascular health.

2. Increased Stamina and Endurance: Engaging in regular cardiovascular exercise boosts your stamina and endurance, allowing you to perform daily activities with less fatigue and greater efficiency. Whether it's climbing stairs, carrying groceries, or playing with your grandchildren, improved endurance makes everyday tasks easier and more enjoyable.

3. Weight Management: Cardiovascular exercise is an effective tool for burning calories and supporting weight loss or weight maintenance. By increasing energy expenditure, cardio helps create a calorie deficit, which is essential for shedding excess pounds and achieving a healthy body weight.

4. Enhanced Mood and Mental Well-being: Cardiovascular exercise triggers the release of endorphins, chemicals in the brain that promote feelings of happiness and reduce stress and anxiety. Regular cardio sessions can boost your mood, alleviate symptoms of depression, and improve overall mental well-being.

5. Better Sleep Quality: Engaging in regular cardiovascular exercise has been linked to improved

sleep quality and duration. Exercise encourages relaxation, eases insomnia symptoms, and helps balance the sleep-wake cycle, all of which contribute to more comfortable and rejuvenating sleep.

6. Reduced Risk of Chronic Diseases: Cardiovascular exercise plays a crucial role in reducing the risk of chronic diseases such as type 2 diabetes, stroke, and certain types of cancer. By improving heart health, controlling blood sugar levels, and promoting healthy weight management, cardio helps protect against various health conditions.

7. Increased Energy Levels: Regular cardiovascular exercise boosts energy levels by enhancing circulation, oxygen delivery, and nutrient uptake throughout the body. Whether it's an early morning jog or a lunchtime swim, starting your day with cardio can invigorate you and set a positive tone for the rest of the day.

Practical Tips for Cardiovascular Exercise

1. Choose Activities You Enjoy: The key to sticking with a cardio routine is finding activities that you enjoy. Whether it's walking in nature, cycling through the park, dancing to your favorite music, or swimming laps in the pool, choose activities that you look forward to and that bring you joy.

2. Start Slowly and Progress Gradually: If you're new to cardiovascular exercise or have been inactive for a while, start with low-impact activities and gradually increase the duration, intensity, and frequency of your workouts. Pay attention to your body's signals and move at a speed that suits you.

3. Mix It Up: Keep your cardio routine interesting and challenging by incorporating a variety of activities into your schedule. Try different forms of cardio, such as walking, running, cycling, swimming, dancing, and group fitness classes, to target different muscle groups and prevent boredom.

4. Set Realistic Goals: Set specific, achievable goals for your cardiovascular exercise routine, whether it's increasing your weekly mileage, improving your pace, or completing a certain number of workouts per week. Setting and maintaining specific goals will help you stay motivated and progress-focused.

5. Schedule Regular Workouts: Treat your cardio workouts like appointments that you can't miss. Schedule them into your calendar at times that work best for you, whether it's first thing in the morning, during your lunch break, or in the evening after work. Consistency is key to reaping the benefits of cardiovascular exercise.

6. Listen to Your Body: Pay attention to how your body responds to cardiovascular exercise and adjust your intensity or duration accordingly. If you experience pain, dizziness, or shortness of breath, stop exercising and rest. It's essential to prioritize safety and avoid overexertion to prevent injury.

7. Warm Up and Cool Down: Always start your cardio workouts with a proper warm-up to prepare your body for exercise and reduce the risk of injury. Incorporate dynamic stretches and light cardio activities, such as walking or jogging, to gradually elevate your heart rate and loosen up your muscles. Similarly, finish your workouts with a cool-down period to help your body recover and return to a resting state.

8. Stay Hydrated and Fuel Your Body: Drink plenty of water before, during, and after your cardio workouts to stay hydrated and maintain optimal performance. Fuel your body with nutritious foods, including carbohydrates for energy and protein for muscle repair and recovery, to support your exercise efforts.

9. Monitor Your Progress: Keep track of your cardio workouts, including the duration, intensity, and type of activity, as well as any changes in how you feel or perform. Tracking your progress can help you

identify patterns, set new goals, and celebrate your achievements along the way.

In conclusion, cardiovascular exercise offers a multitude of benefits for physical, mental, and emotional health. By incorporating regular cardio workouts into your routine and following these practical tips, you can improve heart health, increase stamina, manage weight, boost mood, and reduce the risk of chronic diseases. Whether it's a leisurely stroll or an intense cycling class, find activities that you enjoy and make cardio a regular part of your lifestyle for a happier, healthier you.

CHAPTER 7:
LIFESTYLE MODIFICATIONS

In our quest for better health and well-being, making positive lifestyle modifications is key. Small changes in our daily habits can lead to significant improvements in our overall quality of life. In this chapter, we'll explore various lifestyle modifications that can promote health and vitality. From diet and exercise to stress management and sleep hygiene, we'll provide practical tips to help you implement these changes and achieve your wellness goals.

1. Healthy Eating Habits

Practical Tips:
- Focus on whole, unprocessed foods: Fill your plate with fruits, vegetables, whole grains, lean proteins, and healthy fats to nourish your body with essential nutrients.
- Exercise portion control: To prevent overindulging and preserve a healthy weight, pay attention to portion proportions.
- Limit processed foods and added sugars: Minimize consumption of processed snacks, sugary beverages, and refined carbohydrates, which can contribute to weight gain and health issues.

- Stay hydrated: Drink plenty of water throughout the day to support digestion, hydration, and overall health.
- Practise mindful eating: Slow down and savour each bite, paying attention to hunger and fullness cues to prevent overeating.

2. Regular Physical Activity

Practical Tips:
- Find activities you enjoy: Choose exercises that you genuinely enjoy, whether it's walking, dancing, cycling, or swimming, to make physical activity a sustainable part of your routine.
- Set achievable goals: Start with realistic fitness goals and gradually increase the intensity, duration, and frequency of your workouts as your fitness improves.
- Incorporate variety: Mix up your workouts to prevent boredom and target different muscle groups. Include aerobic exercise, strength training, flexibility exercises, and balance activities for a well-rounded fitness routine.
- Make it social: Exercise with friends, family, or join group fitness classes to stay motivated and accountable.
- Listen to your body: Pay attention to how your body feels during and after exercise, and adjust your intensity or duration as needed to prevent injury and promote recovery.

3. Stress Management

Practical Tips:
- Practise relaxation techniques: Incorporate relaxation techniques such as deep breathing, meditation, yoga, or tai chi into your daily routine to reduce stress and promote calmness.
- Prioritise self-care: Make time for activities that bring you joy and relaxation, whether it's reading, gardening, listening to music, or taking a warm bath.
- Set boundaries: Learn to say no to tasks or commitments that cause excessive stress or overwhelm, and prioritise activities that nourish your well-being.
- Stay connected: Seek support from friends, family, or a therapist, and maintain social connections to alleviate stress and foster a sense of belonging.
- Stay organised: Use planners, to-do lists, or digital apps to organise your tasks and manage your time effectively, reducing stress and overwhelm.

4. Quality Sleep

Practical Tips:
- Establish a bedtime routine: Create a calming bedtime routine to signal to your body that it's time to wind down and prepare for sleep. This could be reading, having a warm bath, or working on relaxation techniques.

- Keep a regular sleep schedule: Even on weekends, go to bed and wake up at the same time each day to help your body's internal clock function properly sleep quality.
- Establish a sleep-friendly environment: Keep your bedroom calm, dark, and cold to promote restful sleep. Invest in a comfortable mattress, pillows, and bedding to enhance sleep comfort.
- Limit screen time before bed: Avoid electronic devices such as smartphones, tablets, and computers at least an hour before bedtime, as the blue light emitted can interfere with melatonin production and disrupt sleep.
- Watch your caffeine intake: Limit caffeine consumption, especially in the afternoon and evening, as it can interfere with sleep quality and duration.

5. Social Connections

Practical Tips:
- Make time for social activities: Schedule regular social activities with friends, family, or community groups to maintain social connections and combat feelings of loneliness or isolation.
- Reach out to others: Initiate contact with friends or family members, even if it's just a phone call, text message, or video chat, to stay connected and show your support.

- Join clubs or groups: Get involved in clubs, organisations, or hobby groups that align with your interests to meet like-minded individuals and build new social connections.
- Volunteer: Engage in volunteer work or community service to connect with others, contribute to meaningful causes, and gain a sense of fulfilment and purpose.
- Be a good listener: Practise active listening and empathy when interacting with others, and offer support and encouragement when needed.

By implementing these lifestyle modifications into your daily routine, you can enhance your health, happiness, and overall well-being. Remember that change takes time and consistency, so be patient with yourself as you work towards your wellness goals. Celebrate your victories along the road, start small, and concentrate on one behavior at a time. With dedication and determination, you can create a healthier and more fulfilling life for yourself.

STRESS MANAGEMENT TECHNIQUES

Life will always involve stress, but how we handle it can have a big impact on our wellbeing. In this chapter, we'll explore various stress management techniques that can help you navigate life's challenges with greater ease and resilience. Drawing from both research-based strategies and personal experiences, we'll delve into practical techniques to cope with stress and cultivate a sense of calm and balance in your life.

Understanding Stress

Stress is your body's natural response to perceived threats or demands, triggering a cascade of physiological and psychological reactions. While some stress can be beneficial, motivating us to take action and adapt to changing circumstances, chronic or excessive stress can take a toll on our health and happiness.

Identifying Personal Stressors

Before diving into stress management techniques, it's essential to identify your personal stressors—the situations, events, or factors that trigger stress in your life. Reflect on past experiences and current challenges to pinpoint specific stressors, whether it's work deadlines, financial worries, relationship issues, or health concerns. Knowing what stresses you out will help you create focused plans to deal with them.

Practical Stress Management Techniques

1. Deep Breathing Exercises

One of the simplest and most effective ways to reduce stress is through deep breathing exercises. Deep breathing activates the body's relaxation response, calming the nervous system and promoting a sense of peace and relaxation. Try the following technique:

- Close your eyes and find a comfortable position, either sitting or lying down.
- Inhale deeply through your nose, filling your lungs with air and expanding your belly.
- Hold your breath for a moment, then exhale slowly and completely through your mouth, releasing tension and stress with each breath.
- Repeat this process for several minutes, focusing on the rhythm of your breath and letting go of any tension or worry with each exhale.

*Personal Experience: When I feel overwhelmed or anxious, I often turn to deep breathing exercises to help me calm my mind and body. Taking a few minutes to focus on my breath allows me to step back from stressful thoughts and regain a sense of balance and clarity.

2. Mindfulness Meditation

Mindfulness meditation involves bringing your attention to the present moment, without judgement or attachment to thoughts or emotions. Practising mindfulness can help reduce stress, anxiety, and rumination, allowing you to cultivate a greater sense of peace and acceptance. Here's how to get started:

- Find a quiet space where you won't be disturbed and sit comfortably with your back straight and your feet flat on the ground.
- Shut your eyes and focus on your breathing, taking note of how each breath feels as you inhale and exhale.
- If your thoughts stray, gently bring them back to your breathing without passing judgment.
- As you continue to practice mindfulness meditation, you may notice a greater sense of calm, clarity, and presence in your daily life.

Personal Experience: Incorporating mindfulness meditation into my daily routine has been transformative in managing stress and enhancing my overall well-being. By taking just a few minutes each day to sit in stillness and observe my breath,

I've learned to navigate challenging situations with greater ease and resilience.

3. Physical Exercise

Exercise is a powerful stress reliever, releasing endorphins and reducing levels of stress hormones in the body. Whether it's a brisk walk, a yoga class, or a dance session, physical activity can help alleviate tension, boost mood, and improve overall well-being. Find enjoyable activities to include into your routine on a regular basis.

Personal Experience: Whenever I'm feeling stressed or overwhelmed, I lace up my sneakers and go for a run in nature. The rhythmic pounding of my feet on the pavement and the fresh air on my face help me clear my mind and release built-up tension, leaving me feeling refreshed and rejuvenated.

4. Healthy Lifestyle Habits

In addition to specific stress management techniques, maintaining a healthy lifestyle can also help reduce stress and promote overall well-being. Be sure to prioritize:

- Healthy Eating: Fuel your body with nutritious foods that nourish and energize you, avoiding excessive caffeine, sugar, and processed foods that can exacerbate stress.

- Adequate Sleep: To promote both physical and mental health, aim for 7-9 hours of good sleep every night. To maximize the quality of your sleep, develop a regular sleep regimen and a calming nighttime ritual.

- Social Support: Cultivate strong social connections with friends, family, and community members who provide support, empathy, and companionship during times of stress.

- Time Management: Break tasks down into manageable steps, set realistic goals, and prioritize your time effectively to reduce feelings of overwhelm and procrastination.

Conclusion

Managing stress is essential for maintaining health, happiness, and overall well-being. By incorporating stress management techniques into your daily routine and making self-care a priority, you can navigate life's challenges with greater ease and resilience. Whether it's deep breathing exercises, mindfulness meditation, physical activity, or healthy lifestyle habits, find what works best for you.

QUALITY SLEEP FOR WEIGHT LOSS

Although it's sometimes disregarded, getting enough sleep is essential for both weight loss and general wellness. In this chapter, we'll explore the connection between sleep and weight loss and provide practical tips to improve sleep quality for better weight management.

Understanding the Link Between Sleep and Weight Loss

Sleep and weight loss are intricately linked, with research consistently showing that insufficient or poor-quality sleep can negatively impact metabolism, appetite regulation, and food choices, ultimately leading to weight gain. Here's how:

1. Metabolism: Sleep deprivation disrupts metabolic hormones, such as leptin and ghrelin, which regulate hunger and satiety. When you don't get enough sleep, leptin levels decrease, signalling hunger, while ghrelin levels increase, promoting appetite. Overeating and weight increase over time may result from this imbalance.

2. Food Cravings: Lack of sleep can increase cravings for high-calorie, carbohydrate-rich foods, such as sweets, salty snacks, and fast food. Sleep deprivation

alters brain activity in areas responsible for food cravings and reward, making it harder to resist unhealthy food choices.

3. Energy Levels: Poor sleep quality can leave you feeling tired, lethargic, and less motivated to engage in physical activity. When you're sleep-deprived, you're more likely to skip workouts and opt for sedentary activities, which can hinder weight loss efforts.

4. Insulin Sensitivity: Sleep deprivation can impair insulin sensitivity, making it harder for your body to regulate blood sugar levels and leading to increased fat storage and weight gain, particularly around the abdominal area.

Practical Tips for Quality Sleep for Weight Loss

1. Create a Regular Sleep Schedule: Even on the weekends, go to bed and wake up at the same time every day. Consistency helps regulate your body's internal clock, improve sleep quality, and promote overall well-being.

2. Create a Relaxing Bedtime Routine: Develop a calming bedtime routine to signal to your body that it's time to wind down and prepare for sleep. This could involve reading, having a warm bath,

meditating, deep breathing, or listening to calming music, among other relaxation techniques.

3. Limit Screen Time Before Bed: Avoid electronic devices such as smartphones, tablets, computers, and televisions at least an hour before bedtime. The blue light emitted by screens can disrupt melatonin production, making it harder to fall asleep and negatively impacting sleep quality.

4. Create a Comfortable Sleep Environment: Make your bedroom conducive to sleep by keeping it cool, dark, quiet, and comfortable. Invest on a comfortable mattress and pillows, block off light with blackout curtains or an eye mask, and reduce noise disturbances with earplugs or white noise generators.

5. Watch Your Caffeine Intake: Limit caffeine consumption, especially in the afternoon and evening, as it can interfere with sleep quality and duration. Opt for decaffeinated beverages or herbal teas in the evening, and avoid stimulants like caffeine and nicotine close to bedtime.

6. Limit Alcohol Consumption: While alcohol may initially make you feel drowsy, it can disrupt sleep patterns and lead to fragmented sleep later in the night. Limit alcohol consumption, particularly in the

hours leading up to bedtime, to improve sleep quality.

7. Exercise Regularly: Engage in regular physical activity, but avoid vigorous exercise close to bedtime, as it can interfere with sleep. Aim for moderate-intensity workouts earlier in the day, which can promote deeper, more restorative sleep at night.

8. Manage Stress: Practice stress management techniques such as deep breathing, meditation, yoga, or progressive muscle relaxation to reduce stress levels and promote relaxation before bedtime. A calm mind and body are essential for quality sleep.

9. Avoid Heavy Meals Before Bed: Avoid large, heavy meals, spicy foods, and caffeine or alcohol close to bedtime, as they can cause indigestion, discomfort, and disrupt sleep. Opt for lighter, easily digestible snacks if you're hungry before bed.

10. Seek Professional Help if Needed: If you continue to struggle with sleep despite implementing these tips, consider seeking help from a healthcare professional. They can evaluate underlying factors contributing to sleep disturbances and recommend personalised treatment options to improve sleep quality.

In conclusion, quality sleep is essential for weight loss and overall health. By prioritising sleep hygiene, establishing a consistent sleep schedule, and practising relaxation techniques, you can improve sleep quality, regulate appetite and metabolism, and support your weight loss efforts. Remember that small changes in your sleep habits can lead to significant improvements in your health and well-being over time.

STRATEGIES FOR SUSTAINABLE WEIGHT LOSS

Achieving and maintaining a healthy weight is a common goal for many people, but it's essential to approach weight loss in a sustainable way to ensure long-term success. In this chapter, we'll explore practical strategies for sustainable weight loss that focus on making healthy lifestyle changes rather than quick fixes or fad diets. By incorporating these strategies into your daily routine, you can achieve lasting results and improve your overall health and well-being.

1. Set Realistic Goals

Achieving long-term weight loss requires setting reasonable and attainable goals.

When dining out, use smaller bowls and plates, calculate serving proportions, and pay attention to portion sizes. Set specific, measurable, and realistic goals, such as losing 1-2 pounds per week or increasing your daily physical activity by 30 minutes. Celebrate small victories along the way and adjust your goals as needed based on your progress and preferences.

2. Adopt a Balanced Diet

A balanced diet is key to sustainable weight loss. Instead of following restrictive diets or cutting out entire food groups, focus on eating a variety of nutrient-dense foods in appropriate portions. Fill your plate with fruits, vegetables, whole grains, lean proteins, and healthy fats, and limit processed foods, sugary beverages, and excessive amounts of added sugars and fats. Practise mindful eating, paying attention to hunger and fullness cues, and savoring each bite to prevent overeating.

3. Practice Portion Control

Controlling portion sizes is essential to managing weight. When ingested in excess, even healthful meals can cause weight gain. Use smaller plates and bowls, measure out serving sizes, and be mindful of portion sizes when dining out. Pay attention to your body's signals of hunger and fullness, and stop eating when you're satisfied but not too full. Eating smaller, more frequent meals throughout the day can also help regulate hunger and prevent overeating.

4. Stay Hydrated

Water consumption should be sufficient for overall health and to help with weight loss. Water helps keep you hydrated, promotes satiety, and may even boost metabolism. Aim to drink at least 8-10 cups of water per day, and choose water as your primary beverage rather than sugary drinks or calorie-laden beverages. Stay hydrated throughout the day, and drink water before meals to help control appetite and prevent overeating.

5. Include Regular Physical Activity

Frequent exercise is crucial for long-term weight loss and good health in general. Aim for two or more days of muscle-strengthening activities in addition to 75 minutes of vigorous-intensity aerobic activity or at least 150 minutes of moderate-intensity aerobic activity each week. Find activities that you enjoy, whether it's walking, swimming, cycling, dancing, or participating in group fitness classes, and make physical activity a regular part of your routine.

6. Prioritise Sleep

Although it is sometimes disregarded, getting enough sleep is essential for controlling weight. Lack of sleep can disrupt hunger hormones, increase cravings for unhealthy foods, and negatively impact metabolism and energy levels. Make sure you get between seven and nine hours of good sleep every night, and stick to a regular sleep routine by going to bed and waking up at the same times every day. To encourage sound sleep, establish a calming nighttime routine, limit screen time before bed, and furnish a cosy sleeping space.

7. Manage Stress

Chronic stress can contribute to weight gain and sabotage weight loss efforts. Practice stress management techniques such as deep breathing, meditation, yoga, or progressive muscle relaxation to reduce stress levels and promote relaxation. Find healthy ways to cope with stress, such as engaging in hobbies, spending time outdoors, or connecting with friends and family. Make self-care a priority and schedule leisure and happy activities.

8. Seek Support

Seeking support from friends, family, or a healthcare professional can enhance your success in achieving sustainable weight loss. Talk to people about your objectives to get their help and inspiration along the way. Consider joining a weight loss support group or working with a registered dietitian or certified personal trainer who can provide guidance, accountability, and personalised recommendations to help you reach your goals.

Conclusion

Sustainable weight loss requires a combination of healthy eating, regular physical activity, adequate sleep, stress management, and support from others. By adopting realistic goals, making gradual lifestyle changes, and focusing on long-term habits rather than short-term fixes, you can achieve lasting results and improve your overall health and well-being. Remember that sustainable weight loss is not about perfection but progress, and every small step forward brings you closer to your goals.

CHAPTER 8:
OVERCOMING CHALLENGES

Life is full of challenges, both big and small, that test our resilience and determination. In this chapter, we'll explore strategies for overcoming challenges and navigating obstacles with grace and perseverance. Drawing from both research-based techniques and personal experiences, we'll delve into practical ways to overcome adversity and emerge stronger on the other side.

Understanding Challenges

Challenges come in many forms, from everyday obstacles like time constraints and financial pressures to major life events such as job loss, illness, or relationship struggles. While challenges can be daunting, they also present opportunities for growth, learning, and personal development. By adopting a positive mindset and implementing effective strategies, we can overcome obstacles and thrive in the face of adversity.

Identifying Personal Challenges

Recognizing and accepting our own troubles is a necessary first step toward successfully overcoming obstacles. Reflect on past experiences and current obstacles to pinpoint the specific challenges you're facing. Whether it's overcoming procrastination, managing stress, navigating career transitions, or coping with personal setbacks, recognizing your challenges is the first step toward finding solutions.

Practical Strategies for Overcoming Challenges

1. Set Clear Goals: Establish clear and achievable goals to guide your actions and keep you focused on the desired outcome. Divide more ambitious objectives into more doable, smaller ones, and acknowledge your progress as you go. Having a clear sense of direction can provide motivation and clarity, making it easier to overcome obstacles.

Personal Experience: When I faced a significant career transition, I set specific goals for updating my skills, networking with industry professionals, and exploring new opportunities. By breaking down my larger goal into actionable steps, I felt more empowered and motivated to navigate the challenges ahead.

2. Develop Resilience: Resilience is the ability to bounce back from adversity and adapt to change. Cultivate resilience by reframing negative thoughts, practising self-compassion, and maintaining a positive outlook in the face of setbacks. Focus on your strengths and past successes, and remind

yourself that challenges are opportunities for growth
and learning.

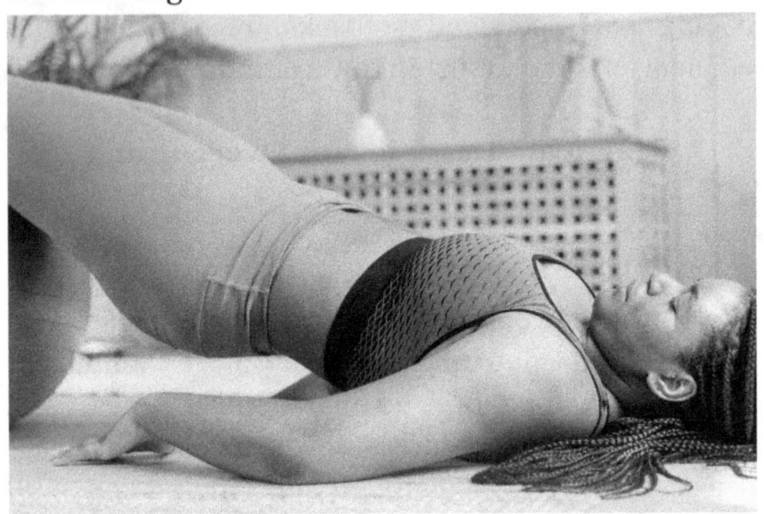

Personal Experience: During a period of personal loss, I leaned on my support network and practised self-care to build resilience. By acknowledging my emotions, seeking support from loved ones, and focusing on small victories, I was able to navigate the challenges with greater strength and resilience.

3. Seek Support: Don't hesitate to reach out for support from friends, family, or professionals when facing challenges. Surround yourself with people who uplift and encourage you, and lean on their support during difficult times. Whether it's seeking advice, venting frustrations, or simply receiving a listening ear, support from others can make a significant difference in overcoming challenges.

Personal Experience: When I struggled with overwhelming stress, I sought support from a therapist who provided guidance and coping strategies. Having a safe space to express my thoughts and feelings allowed me to gain clarity and perspective, ultimately helping me overcome the challenges I faced.

4. Take Action: Instead of dwelling on the challenges you face, take proactive steps to address them head-on. Break tasks down into manageable steps, prioritise your actions, and take consistent action toward finding solutions. By taking control of your circumstances and focusing on what you can change,

you'll feel empowered to overcome obstacles and move forward.

Personal Experience: When I encountered financial difficulties, I took proactive steps to assess my budget, explore additional income opportunities, and seek financial assistance where needed. By taking action and staying focused on solutions, I was able to overcome the challenges and regain financial stability.

5. Practice Self-Care: Self-care is essential for maintaining mental, emotional, and physical well-being, especially during challenging times. Make time for activities that nourish and recharge you, whether it's exercise, meditation, spending time in nature, or engaging in hobbies you enjoy. Prioritise self-care as a way to replenish your energy and resilience.

Personal Experience: During a period of burnout, I prioritised self-care by incorporating daily walks in nature, practising mindfulness meditation, and setting boundaries around work commitments. By making self-care a non-negotiable part of my routine, I was better equipped to face the challenges ahead with a renewed sense of energy and perspective.

Conclusion

Challenges are an inevitable part of life, but they don't have to define us. By adopting a proactive mindset, seeking support, and implementing practical strategies, we can overcome obstacles and emerge stronger on the other side. Remember that challenges are opportunities for growth and learning, and every obstacle you overcome brings you one step closer to achieving your goals and living your best life.

DEALING WITH PLATEAUS

Plateaus are a common occurrence in various aspects of life, from weight loss and fitness progress to career advancement and personal growth. In this chapter, we'll explore what plateaus are, why they happen, and most importantly, practical strategies for overcoming them. Whether you're striving to lose weight, improve your fitness, or achieve success in other areas of your life, understanding how to navigate plateaus is essential for continued progress and success.

Understanding Plateaus

A plateau is a period of stagnant progress or a temporary halt in improvement despite consistent efforts. Plateaus can be frustrating and disheartening, causing individuals to feel stuck or demotivated. However, plateaus are a natural part of the process, and experiencing them does not mean failure. Instead, plateaus provide an opportunity for reflection, adjustment, and renewed focus to push past obstacles and continue moving forward.

Why Plateaus Happen

Plateaus can occur for various reasons, depending on the context. In the realm of weight loss and fitness, plateaus often occur due to:

1. Adaptation: The body adapts to changes in diet and exercise over time, leading to a slowdown in weight loss or muscle gain.

2. Metabolic Changes: As weight decreases, the body's metabolic rate may decrease, requiring fewer calories to maintain weight loss.

3. Lack of Variety: Repeating the same workouts or following the same dietary patterns can lead to a plateau as the body becomes accustomed to the routine.

4. Stress and Hormones: Stress, lack of sleep, and hormonal fluctuations can impact weight loss progress by affecting appetite, metabolism, and energy levels.

Practical Tips for Dealing with Plateaus

1. Reassess Your Goals: Take a step back and reassess your goals to ensure they are realistic, achievable, and aligned with your current priorities and values. Adjust your goals if necessary to reflect your evolving needs and circumstances.

2. Track Your Progress: Keep track of your food intake, exercise routine, and other relevant metrics to identify patterns and trends over time. Monitoring your progress can help you pinpoint areas where you may need to make adjustments.

3. Modify Your Exercise Routine: Shake up your workout routine by incorporating new exercises, changing the intensity or duration of your workouts, or trying different forms of exercise altogether. Cross-training can help prevent boredom, challenge different muscle groups, and stimulate further progress.

4. Adjust Your Nutrition Plan: Review your dietary habits and make adjustments as needed to break through a weight loss plateau. Focus on nutrient-dense foods, adjust portion sizes if necessary, and consider consulting with a registered dietitian for personalised guidance.

5. Increase Activity Levels: Look for opportunities to increase your overall activity levels throughout the day, such as taking the stairs instead of the elevator, going for walks during breaks, or incorporating more movement into your daily routine. Non-exercise physical activity can contribute to calorie expenditure and support weight loss efforts.

6. Prioritise Sleep and Stress Management: Ensure you're getting adequate sleep and managing stress effectively, as these factors can impact weight loss progress. Aim for 7-9 hours of quality sleep per night and incorporate stress-reduction techniques such as meditation, deep breathing, or yoga into your routine.

7. Stay Consistent and Patient: Plateaus are a natural part of the process, and it's essential to stay consistent with your efforts and patient with the process. Trust in your ability to overcome obstacles and focus on making sustainable lifestyle changes rather than seeking quick fixes or drastic measures.

8. Seek Support and Accountability: Reach out to friends, family, or a support group for encouragement and accountability during challenging times. Having a support system can provide motivation, perspective, and guidance as you navigate through plateaus and setbacks.

Conclusion

Plateaus are a normal and expected part of any journey toward improvement and success. By understanding why plateaus happen and implementing practical strategies to overcome them, you can break through obstacles, regain momentum, and continue making progress toward your goals. Remember to stay flexible, adaptable, and resilient in the face of challenges, and celebrate your victories, no matter how small, along the way. With perseverance and determination, you can overcome plateaus and achieve the success you desire.

HANDLING EMOTIONAL EATING

Emotional eating is a common phenomenon that many of us experience at some point in our lives. It's when we turn to food not because we're physically hungry, but because we're seeking comfort, distraction, or relief from difficult emotions. In this chapter, we'll explore what emotional eating is, why it happens, and most importantly, how to manage it effectively.

Understanding Emotional Eating:

Imagine this scenario: You've had a stressful day at work. Your boss criticised your performance, your inbox is overflowing with unanswered emails, and you're feeling overwhelmed. As you walk through the door of your home, you head straight to the kitchen and reach for a bag of chips. Sound familiar? That's emotional eating in action.

Emotions such as stress, anxiety, depression, boredom, or even happiness can set off emotional eating. It's a way to cope with emotions that feel too overwhelming to handle. When we eat in response to emotions rather than hunger, we're not addressing the root cause of our feelings. Instead, we're using food as a temporary Band-Aid.

My Experience:

I remember a time when I used to turn to food whenever I felt stressed or anxious. Whether it was a looming deadline or a disagreement with a loved one, I found solace in sugary snacks and comfort foods. However, I soon realised that this pattern only left me feeling worse in the long run. Not only did I not address the underlying issues, but I also began to feel guilty and ashamed of my eating habits.

Recognizing Triggers:

Knowing what your triggers are is one of the first steps towards controlling your emotional eating. What emotions or situations tend to lead you to the kitchen? Is it boredom? Loneliness? Stress? By identifying your triggers, you can begin to develop healthier coping mechanisms.

For example, if you find that you often reach for snacks when you're bored, try finding alternative activities to keep yourself occupied. Take a walk outside, call a friend, or try a new hobby. By engaging in activities that fulfil you in other ways, you'll be less likely to turn to food for comfort.

Developing Coping Strategies:

Once you've identified your triggers, it's time to develop coping strategies that don't involve food. This could include practising relaxation techniques such as deep breathing or meditation, journaling your thoughts and feelings, or seeking support from a therapist or support group.

In my personal experience, I discovered that regulating my emotional eating was much aided by engaging in mindfulness practices. By staying present in the moment and paying attention to my thoughts and feelings without judgment, I was better able to respond to them in a healthy way.

Building a Support System:

Finally, don't be afraid to reach out for support. Whether it's friends, family, or a professional therapist, having a support system in place can make all the difference in overcoming emotional eating. Surround yourself with people who understand your struggles and are willing to offer encouragement and guidance along the way.

Conclusion:

In conclusion, emotional eating is a common but manageable issue that many of us face. By understanding our triggers, developing healthy coping strategies, and building a support system, we can learn to overcome emotional eating and establish a healthier relationship with food.
Recall that every step you take to control your emotional eating is a step toward a happier, healthier you, and that it's acceptable to ask for assistance when necessary.

COPING WITH SOCIAL PRESSURES

In today's world, social pressures are everywhere. Whether it's feeling the need to fit in with a certain group, live up to society's expectations, or constantly compare ourselves to others on social media, navigating these pressures can be challenging. But fear not, in this chapter, we'll explore practical tips for coping with social pressures in a healthy and constructive way.

Understanding Social Pressures:

Social pressures can come from various sources, including peers, family, media, and even our own internal expectations. They can manifest in different ways, such as feeling the need to conform to certain standards of appearance, behaviour, or success. These pressures can be both overt and subtle, but their impact on our mental and emotional well-being can be significant.

My Experience:

Growing up, I often felt pressure to excel academically, look a certain way, and fit in with the popular crowd. It wasn't until later in life that I realised the toll these pressures were taking on my self-esteem and happiness. Through trial and error,

I've learned effective strategies for coping with social pressures, and I'm here to share them with you.

Practical Tips for Coping with Social Pressures:

1. Define Your Values:

 Think on your values and the things that are really important to you for a while.
What are your priorities in life? By having a clear understanding of your values, you can better navigate social pressures and make decisions that align with your authentic self.

2. Set Boundaries:

Learn to set boundaries with others and assertively communicate your needs and limits. It's okay to say no to things that don't align with your values or make you uncomfortable. Remember, your well-being is important, and it's okay to prioritise it.

3. Practice Self-Compassion:

Be kind to yourself and practice self-compassion. Remember that nobody is perfect, and it's okay to make mistakes or fall short of expectations sometimes. Show yourself the same consideration and compassion that you would extend to a friend in a comparable circumstance.

4. Limit Social Media Usage:

While social media can be a great way to stay connected, it can also exacerbate feelings of inadequacy and comparison. Consider limiting your social media usage or taking breaks when you feel overwhelmed. Remember that people often only show the highlight reels of their lives online, and it's not an accurate representation of reality.

5. Surround Yourself with Supportive People:

 Be in the company of positive, affirming individuals who value and embrace you for who you are. Cultivate relationships with friends, family, or mentors who accept you unconditionally and encourage you to be your authentic self. Having a strong support system can help buffer against social pressures and provide a sense of belonging and validation.

6. Focus on Personal Growth:

Instead of constantly comparing yourself to others, focus on your own personal growth and development. Make significant goals for yourself and progress toward them at your own speed. Honor your accomplishments, no matter how modest, and recognize the strides you've made in the process.

Conclusion:

In conclusion, coping with social pressures is an ongoing journey that requires self-awareness, resilience, and self-compassion. By defining your values, setting boundaries, practicing self-compassion, limiting social media usage, surrounding yourself with supportive people, and focusing on personal growth, you can navigate social pressures in a healthy and constructive way. Remember, you are worthy and deserving of love and acceptance just as you are.

CHAPTER 9:
SPECIAL CONSIDERATIONS

As we navigate life, there are certain special considerations that may arise, requiring us to approach situations with care and thoughtfulness. In this chapter, we'll explore practical tips for handling these special considerations in a way that promotes understanding, inclusivity, and compassion.

Navigating Disabilities:

One special consideration to keep in mind is how to navigate interactions with individuals who have disabilities. Whether it's physical, sensory, intellectual, or mental health-related disabilities, it's important to approach these interactions with empathy and respect.

Practical Tips:

1. Use Person-First Language: When referring to individuals with disabilities, use person-first language that emphasises the person rather than the disability. Say "person with a disability" instead of "disabled person," for instance.

2. Ask Before Offering Assistance: If you encounter someone who appears to need assistance due to a

disability, always ask before offering help. Respect their autonomy and allow them to accept or decline assistance as they see fit.

3. Be Patient and Understanding: Individuals with disabilities may require more time or assistance to complete certain tasks. Be patient and understanding, and avoid making assumptions about their abilities or limitations.

4. Accessibility Matters: Consider the accessibility of your environment and make accommodations as needed to ensure that individuals with disabilities can fully participate. This may include providing ramps, elevators, accessible restrooms, and alternative formats for information.

5. Focus on Abilities, Not Limitations: Instead of focusing on what someone with a disability cannot do, focus on their abilities and strengths. They should be treated with the same decency and respect as everyone else.

Navigating Diversity and Inclusion:

Another special consideration to be mindful of is how to navigate diversity and inclusion in various settings, whether it's in the workplace, educational institutions, or within communities.

Practical Tips:

1. Educate Yourself: Take the time to educate yourself about different cultures, backgrounds, and identities. Be open to learning from others and seek out diverse perspectives and experiences.

2. Foster Inclusive Spaces: Create environments that are inclusive and welcoming to people from all backgrounds. Encourage diversity in leadership positions, provide opportunities for underrepresented groups, and actively challenge discrimination and bias.

3. Practise Active Listening: Listen actively and empathetically to the experiences and perspectives of others. Validate their feelings and avoid invalidating or dismissing their experiences.

4. Be an Ally: Stand up for and support marginalised groups, even if you're not directly affected by the issues they face. Use your privilege and influence to advocate for equity and justice.

5. Challenge Stereotypes and Microaggressions: Be aware of your own biases and challenge stereotypes and microaggressions when you encounter them. Speak up against discriminatory language or behaviour and strive to create a culture of respect and acceptance.

Navigating Life Transitions:

Life is full of transitions, both big and small, that can present unique challenges and opportunities for growth. Whether it's starting a new job, moving to a new city, getting married, or becoming a parent, navigating these transitions requires adaptability and resilience.

Practical Tips:

1. Accept Change: Accept change as a chance for personal development and exploration rather than fighting it. Be open to new experiences and challenges, and approach them with a positive mindset.

2. Seek Support: During times of transition, don't be afraid to lean on your support system for guidance and encouragement. Reach out to friends, family, or mentors who can offer advice and support as you navigate the changes.

3. Take Care of Yourself: Self-care is crucial during times of transition. Make sure to prioritise your physical, emotional, and mental well-being by practising self-care activities that nourish and rejuvenate you.

4. Set Realistic Expectations: Be realistic about what you can accomplish during times of transition and don't put too much pressure on yourself to have everything figured out right away. Allow yourself time to adjust and adapt to the changes.

5. Focus on the Positive: While transitions can be challenging, they also offer opportunities for growth and new beginnings. Focus on the positive aspects of the transition and celebrate the progress you've made along the way.

Conclusion:

In conclusion, navigating special considerations requires empathy, understanding, and a willingness to learn and grow. Whether it's interacting with individuals with disabilities, fostering diversity and inclusion, or navigating life transitions, approaching these situations with compassion and respect can lead to more positive and inclusive outcomes for everyone involved. Remember, we are all on this journey together, and by supporting and uplifting one another, we can create a more inclusive and compassionate world.

MENOPAUSE AND WEIGHT LOSS

The end of a woman's reproductive years is marked by the normal biological process of menopause. It typically occurs in women in their late 40s or early 50s, although the exact age varies from person to person. Along with hormonal changes, menopause can also bring about changes in metabolism and body composition, making weight management a common concern for many women during this stage of life. In this chapter, we'll explore practical tips for managing weight during menopause in a healthy and sustainable way.

Understanding Menopause and Weight Gain:

During menopause, a woman's body undergoes several hormonal changes, including a decrease in estrogen levels. These hormonal changes can lead to a slowing of the metabolism, an increase in abdominal fat, and a redistribution of body fat from the hips and thighs to the abdomen. These changes can contribute to weight gain and make it more challenging to lose weight.

Practical Tips for Weight Loss During Menopause:

1. Focus on Nutrition:

Eating a balanced diet is essential for managing weight during menopause. Make a point of including a lot of nutritious grains, fruits, veggies, lean meats, and healthy fats in your meals. Avoid highly processed foods, sugary snacks, and excessive amounts of alcohol, which can contribute to weight gain.

2. Pay Attention to Portion Sizes:

During menopause, it's important to pay attention to portion sizes and avoid overeating. Use smaller plates and bowls to help control portion sizes, and try to eat mindfully, paying attention to hunger and fullness cues.

3. Stay Active:

Regular physical activity is key for managing weight during menopause. Aim for two or more days of muscle-strengthening exercises per week in addition to at least 150 minutes of moderate-intensity activity or 75 minutes of vigorous-intensity exercise every week. Find activities that you enjoy, whether it's walking, swimming, yoga, or dancing, and make them a regular part of your routine.

4. Incorporate Strength Training:

In addition to aerobic exercise, incorporating strength training into your routine can help maintain muscle mass and boost metabolism during menopause. Focus on exercises that target major muscle groups, such as squats, lunges, push-ups, and planks, and gradually increase the intensity and duration as you build strength.

5. Prioritise Sleep:

Getting enough sleep is crucial for managing weight during menopause. Aim for seven to nine hours of quality sleep per night, and establish a regular sleep schedule to help regulate your body's internal clock. Avoid caffeine, nicotine, and electronics before bedtime, and create a relaxing bedtime routine to help signal to your body that it's time to wind down.

6. Manage Stress:

Chronic stress can contribute to weight gain and make it more difficult to lose weight during menopause. Practice stress-reduction techniques such as deep breathing, meditation, yoga, or spending time in nature to help manage stress levels and promote overall well-being.

7. Seek Support:

Navigating weight loss during menopause can be challenging, so don't be afraid to seek support from friends, family, or a healthcare professional. Consider joining a support group or enlisting the help of a registered dietitian or personal trainer who can provide guidance and accountability along the way.

Conclusion:

In conclusion, managing weight during menopause requires a combination of healthy eating, regular exercise, adequate sleep, stress management, and social support. By adopting these practical tips and making lifestyle changes that promote overall health and well-being, you can successfully navigate weight loss during menopause and feel your best at every stage of life. Remember, it's never too late to prioritise your health and make positive changes that support your long-term well-being.

HEALTH CONDITIONS AND WEIGHT MANAGEMENT

Maintaining a healthy weight is important for overall well-being, but for many people, managing weight can be challenging, especially when dealing with underlying health conditions. In this chapter, we'll explore the relationship between health conditions and weight management, and provide practical tips for navigating this complex interplay.

Understanding Health Conditions and Weight Management:

Health conditions can have a significant impact on weight management, both directly and indirectly. Certain conditions, such as thyroid disorders, polycystic ovary syndrome (PCOS), diabetes, and hormonal imbalances, can affect metabolism, appetite regulation, and energy levels, making it more difficult to lose weight. Additionally, medications used to treat these conditions may also contribute to weight gain or make weight loss efforts more challenging.

My Experience:

I've personally struggled with managing my weight while dealing with health conditions such as hypothyroidism and insulin resistance. Despite my best efforts to eat healthily and exercise regularly, I found it difficult to lose weight and maintain a healthy BMI. However, through trial and error, I've learned effective strategies for managing my weight while navigating these health challenges.

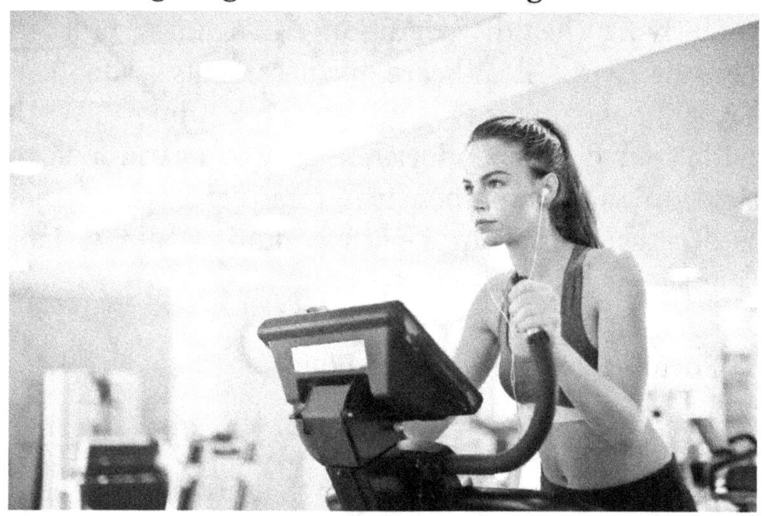

Practical Tips for Weight Management with Health Conditions:

1. Consult with Healthcare Professionals:

If you're struggling to manage your weight due to underlying health conditions, it's important to consult with healthcare professionals who can provide personalised guidance and support. Work with your doctor, endocrinologist, or nutritionist to develop a comprehensive treatment plan that addresses both your health condition and weight management goals.

2. Focus on Nutrient-Dense Foods:

When managing weight with health conditions, prioritise nutrient-dense foods that provide essential vitamins, minerals, and antioxidants to support overall health and well-being. Aim to fill your plate with plenty of fruits, vegetables, whole grains, lean proteins, and healthy fats, and limit processed foods, sugary snacks, and refined carbohydrates.

3. Monitor Portion Sizes:

Pay attention to portion sizes and be mindful of your calorie intake, especially if you're taking medications that may affect appetite or metabolism. Use measuring cups, food scales, or visual cues to help control portion sizes, and avoid mindless eating or emotional eating habits that can contribute to weight gain.

4. Stay Active within Your Limits:

Regular physical activity is important for managing weight and promoting overall health, but it's essential to find activities that are appropriate for your health condition and fitness level. Whether it's walking, swimming, cycling, or yoga, choose activities that you enjoy and can safely participate in without exacerbating symptoms or causing injury.

5. Monitor Medication Effects:

Be aware of how medications used to treat health conditions may affect weight and metabolism. Some medications may cause weight gain as a side effect, while others may suppress appetite or alter nutrient absorption. Discuss any concerns or changes in weight with your healthcare provider, and explore alternative treatment options if necessary.

6. Practise Mindful Eating:

Practise mindful eating techniques to help regulate appetite, promote satiety, and prevent overeating. Pay attention to hunger and fullness cues, eat slowly and savour each bite, and avoid distractions such as television or electronic devices during meals. By tuning into your body's signals, you can better regulate food intake and support weight management goals.

7. Seek Support and Accountability:

Navigating weight management with health conditions can be challenging, so don't hesitate to seek support from friends, family, or support groups who understand your struggles and can offer encouragement and accountability. Consider joining online communities or forums where you can connect with others facing similar challenges and share experiences and strategies for success.

Conclusion:

In conclusion, managing weight with health conditions requires a personalised approach that takes into account the unique challenges and considerations of each individual. By consulting with healthcare professionals, focusing on nutrient-dense foods, monitoring portion sizes, staying active within your limits, monitoring medication effects, practising mindful eating, and seeking support and accountability, you can successfully navigate weight management while prioritising your health and well-being. Remember, progress may be slow and setbacks may occur, but with perseverance and determination, you can achieve your weight management goals.

STRATEGIES FOR BUSY WOMEN

As a busy woman juggling multiple responsibilities, finding time for self-care, health, and personal development can often feel like an uphill battle. However, with the right strategies in place, it's possible to effectively manage your time and prioritise your well-being amidst the chaos of daily life. In this chapter, we'll explore practical tips and strategies for busy women to maintain balance, enhance productivity, and foster overall well-being.

1. Prioritise Self-Care:

Self-care is essential for maintaining physical, mental, and emotional well-being, especially when you're constantly on the go. Make self-care a non-negotiable part of your routine by scheduling time for activities that recharge and rejuvenate you. Whether it's taking a long bath, reading a book, practising yoga, or simply enjoying a quiet cup of tea, find activities that nourish your soul and make them a priority.

2. Practice Time Management:

Effective time management is key for busy women to juggle multiple responsibilities and commitments. Start by creating a daily or weekly schedule that outlines your tasks and priorities, and be realistic about how much time you have available for each. Break larger tasks into smaller, manageable chunks, and prioritise your most important tasks first. Consider using productivity tools or apps to help you stay organised and on track.

3. Set Boundaries:

Setting boundaries is crucial for maintaining balance and preventing burnout, especially when you're constantly pulled in multiple directions. Learn to say no to requests or commitments that don't align with your priorities or values, and don't be afraid to delegate tasks or ask for help when needed. Establishing clear boundaries with work, family, and social commitments will help you preserve your time and energy for what truly matters.

4. Streamline Your Routine:

Simplify your daily routine to minimise stress and maximise efficiency. Look for ways to streamline tasks and eliminate unnecessary steps, whether it's meal prepping on weekends, setting up automatic bill payments, or organising your workspace for optimal productivity. By reducing decision fatigue and creating systems that work for you, you'll free up more time and energy for the things that bring you joy.

5. Practice Mindfulness:

Mindfulness is the practice of being fully present in the moment, without judgement or distraction. Incorporate mindfulness into your daily routine by taking short breaks throughout the day to check in with yourself, practise deep breathing or meditation, or simply observe your thoughts and feelings without getting caught up in them. Cultivating mindfulness can help reduce stress, improve focus and concentration, and enhance overall well-being.

6. Stay Active:

Regular physical activity is essential for maintaining health and vitality, even when you're short on time. Find creative ways to incorporate exercise into your busy schedule, whether it's taking the stairs instead of the elevator, going for a walk during your lunch break, or doing quick workouts at home. Aim for at least 30 minutes of moderate-intensity exercise most days of the week, and prioritise activities that you enjoy and can sustain long-term.

7. Foster Supportive Relationships:

Strong social connections are crucial for emotional well-being and resilience, especially during busy and challenging times. Make time for meaningful connections with friends, family, and loved ones, whether it's scheduling regular phone calls or coffee dates, joining a support group or community organisation, or simply reaching out to someone for a quick chat. Surrounding yourself with supportive people who understand and uplift you can provide a valuable source of comfort, encouragement, and perspective.

Conclusion:

In conclusion, being a busy woman doesn't mean sacrificing your health, happiness, or personal fulfilment. By implementing practical strategies for self-care, time management, boundary-setting, routine streamlining, mindfulness, physical activity, and fostering supportive relationships, you can effectively manage your time and priorities while nurturing your overall well-being. Remember, it's okay to prioritise yourself and your needs, and small, consistent actions can lead to meaningful and sustainable change over time.

CHAPTER 10:
TRACKING PROGRESS

Tracking progress is an essential aspect of achieving any goal, whether it's improving your health, building a business, or mastering a new skill. By monitoring your progress regularly, you can identify areas of improvement, stay motivated, and make necessary adjustments to stay on track towards your goals. In this chapter, we'll explore practical tips for tracking progress effectively and efficiently.

1. Set Clear Goals:

Before you can track your progress, it's important to establish clear and specific goals. Whether your goal is to lose weight, save money, or learn a new language, be specific about what you want to achieve and establish measurable criteria for success. For example, instead of setting a vague goal like "lose weight," set a specific goal like "lose 10 pounds in three months."

2. Choose the Right Metrics:

Once you've set your goals, identify the key metrics or indicators that you'll use to track your progress. These metrics will depend on your specific goal but should be objective, measurable, and relevant to your desired outcomes. For example, if your goal is to improve your fitness, you might track metrics like weight, body measurements, exercise duration, and strength gains.

3. Use Tracking Tools:

There are numerous tools and resources available to help you track your progress effectively. Whether it's a simple spreadsheet, a mobile app, or a specialised tracking device, find a tracking tool that works for you and fits your needs. Choose a tool that is easy to use, provides relevant data, and allows you to visualise your progress over time.

4. Establish a Tracking Routine:

Consistency is key when it comes to tracking progress. Establish a regular routine for tracking your metrics, whether it's daily, weekly, or monthly, and stick to it. Set aside dedicated time in your schedule to review your progress, update your tracking tool, and reflect on your accomplishments and areas for improvement.

5. Celebrate Small Wins:

Tracking progress isn't just about reaching your ultimate goal; it's also about celebrating the small wins along the way. Acknowledge and celebrate your progress, no matter how small, to stay motivated and maintain momentum towards your larger goals. Whether it's hitting a new personal record in the gym, saving a certain amount of money, or mastering a difficult skill, take time to acknowledge your achievements and pat yourself on the back.

6. Reflect and Adjust:

Regularly review your progress and reflect on what's working well and what could be improved. Are you making steady progress towards your goals, or are you falling behind? Are there any patterns or trends in your data that you can identify? Use this information to make necessary adjustments to your approach, whether it's tweaking your strategies, setting new goals, or seeking additional support or resources.

7. Stay Flexible:

While it's important to set clear goals and establish a tracking routine, it's also essential to remain flexible and adaptable as circumstances change. Due to the unpredictability of life, challenges and setbacks are unavoidable. Instead of getting discouraged when things don't go as planned, use setbacks as opportunities to learn and grow. Stay flexible in your approach, and be willing to adjust your goals and strategies as needed to stay on course.

8. Seek Accountability and Support:

Having accountability and support can significantly enhance your ability to track progress and achieve your goals. Whether it's a friend, family member, mentor, or coach, share your goals and progress with someone who can hold you accountable and provide encouragement and support along the way. Consider joining a support group or community of like-minded individuals who can offer guidance, motivation, and accountability as you work towards your goals.

Conclusion:

In conclusion, tracking progress is a critical component of goal achievement and personal development. By setting clear goals, choosing the right metrics, using tracking tools, establishing a tracking routine, celebrating small wins, reflecting and adjusting, staying flexible, and seeking accountability and support, you can effectively monitor your progress and stay on track towards your goals. Remember, progress may not always be linear, but with consistency, determination, and a willingness to learn and adapt, you can make meaningful strides towards achieving your goals and creating the life you desire.

IMPORTANCE OF MONITORING

Monitoring is the process of systematically observing and tracking progress, performance, or changes over time. Whether it's monitoring your health, finances, business metrics, or personal goals, monitoring plays a crucial role in achieving success and maintaining accountability. In this chapter, we'll explore the importance of monitoring and provide practical tips for implementing effective monitoring strategies in various aspects of life.

1. Identifying Progress and Success:

One of the primary benefits of monitoring is that it allows you to identify progress and success towards your goals. By tracking relevant metrics and indicators, you can see how far you've come and celebrate your achievements along the way. Whether it's hitting a fitness milestone, reaching a savings target, or achieving a business objective, monitoring helps you recognize your progress and stay motivated to continue moving forward.

2. Detecting Early Warning Signs:

Monitoring also helps you detect early warning signs of potential problems or setbacks before they escalate into larger issues. By regularly reviewing data and performance metrics, you can identify trends, patterns, or anomalies that may indicate underlying problems or challenges. Whether it's a decline in health indicators, a decrease in revenue, or a shift in market trends, early detection allows you to take proactive measures to address issues before they become more significant.

3. Making Informed Decisions:

Effective monitoring provides you with the information and insights needed to make informed decisions about your actions and strategies. Whether it's adjusting your approach, reallocating resources, or pivoting in a new direction, monitoring helps you base decisions on objective data rather than guesswork or intuition. By having a clear understanding of your current status and progress, you can make decisions that are more likely to lead to positive outcomes and success.

4. Maintaining Accountability:

Monitoring holds you accountable for your actions and commitments by providing a tangible record of your progress and performance. When you know that your actions are being tracked and evaluated, you're more likely to stay focused, motivated, and accountable for your goals. Whether it's keeping a food diary to track your eating habits, logging your workouts to monitor your fitness progress, or reviewing your financial statements to track your spending, monitoring keeps you responsible for your actions and your objectives.

5. Improving Efficiency and Effectiveness:

Monitoring allows you to identify areas of inefficiency or ineffectiveness in your processes, strategies, or behaviours and make necessary adjustments to improve performance. By tracking key performance indicators and analysing data, you can identify bottlenecks, streamline workflows, and optimise resources to enhance efficiency and effectiveness. Whether it's identifying time-wasting activities, refining marketing strategies, or streamlining operations, monitoring helps you identify opportunities for improvement and make targeted interventions to achieve better results.

6. Building Habits and Consistency:

Monitoring helps you build habits and consistency by providing a structure for tracking your behaviours and progress over time. Whether it's establishing a daily routine, sticking to an exercise plan, or practising financial discipline, regular monitoring reinforces positive behaviours and habits by holding you accountable and providing feedback on your progress. By consistently tracking your actions and behaviours, you can build momentum, establish new habits, and make lasting changes that contribute to your long-term success and well-being.

7. Enhancing Motivation and Focus:

Finally, monitoring enhances motivation and focus by providing tangible evidence of your progress and accomplishments. When you can see the results of your efforts reflected in the data, you're more likely to stay motivated and focused on your goals. Whether it's seeing improvements in your health metrics, witnessing growth in your savings account, or achieving milestones in your business, monitoring reinforces your efforts and provides a sense of accomplishment that fuels further progress and success.

Conclusion:

In conclusion, monitoring is a critical component of achieving success and maintaining accountability in various aspects of life. By tracking progress, identifying early warning signs, making informed decisions, maintaining accountability, improving efficiency and effectiveness, building habits and consistency, and enhancing motivation and focus, monitoring helps you achieve your goals and realise your full potential. Whether it's monitoring your health, finances, business metrics, or personal goals, implementing effective monitoring strategies can lead to better outcomes, greater success, and a more fulfilling life overall.

KEEPING A FOOD DIARY

Keeping a food diary is a simple yet powerful tool for improving your eating habits, managing your weight, and promoting overall health and well-being. By tracking what you eat and drink, you can gain valuable insights into your dietary patterns, identify areas for improvement, and make informed choices about your nutrition. In this chapter, we'll explore practical tips for keeping a food diary effectively and efficiently.

1. Get Started:

To begin keeping a food diary, all you need is a notebook, journal, or mobile app where you can record your daily food intake. Choose a format that works best for you, whether it's pen and paper or a digital platform, and commit to using it consistently. Remember, the goal is to accurately record everything you eat and drink throughout the day, so be honest and thorough in your tracking.

2. Record Everything:

When keeping a food diary, it's essential to record everything you eat and drink, including portion sizes and any condiments or sauces used. Be as specific as possible when describing your meals and snacks, noting ingredients, cooking methods, and serving sizes. Don't forget to include beverages, snacks, and any extras like sugar or cream in your coffee. The more detailed your entries, the more accurate your food diary will be.

3. Be Consistent:

Consistency is key when it comes to keeping a food diary. Aim to record your food intake shortly after each meal or snack to ensure accuracy and prevent forgetfulness. Set aside a few minutes each day to update your food diary, whether it's after meals, at the end of the day, or first thing in the morning. By making food tracking a regular part of your routine, you'll develop the habit and maintain consistency over time.

4. Include Portion Sizes:

In addition to listing the foods you eat, be sure to include portion sizes in your food diary. Use measuring cups, food scales, or visual cues to estimate portion sizes accurately, and record them in your diary. Pay attention to serving sizes listed on food labels, and be mindful of portion distortion, where serving sizes may be larger than you realise. By accurately tracking portion sizes, you'll have a better understanding of your calorie intake and can make adjustments as needed.

5. Note Hunger and Fullness:

In addition to recording what you eat, consider noting your hunger and fullness levels before and after meals in your food diary. Use a simple scale, such as 1-10, to rate your hunger and fullness levels, with 1 being extremely hungry and 10 being overly full. This can help you become more aware of your eating patterns and identify times when you may be eating out of boredom, stress, or other emotional triggers rather than true hunger.

6. Be Mindful of Eating Context:

When recording your food intake, pay attention to the context in which you eat, including your surroundings, emotions, and triggers. Note any situations or emotions that may influence your eating choices, such as stress, boredom, social gatherings, or emotional eating. By becoming more aware of your eating triggers, you can develop strategies to address them and make healthier choices in the future.

7. Review and Reflect:

Regularly review your food diary to identify patterns, trends, or areas for improvement in your eating habits. Look for opportunities to make healthier choices, such as increasing your intake of fruits and vegetables, reducing portion sizes, or cutting back on sugary snacks and beverages. Reflect on your eating behaviours and consider how they align with your health and wellness goals. Use your food diary as a tool for self-awareness and self-improvement, rather than judgement or criticism.

8. Seek Support:

If you find it challenging to keep a food diary on your own, consider seeking support from a registered dietitian, nutritionist, or health coach who can provide guidance and accountability. They can help you interpret your food diary data, identify areas for improvement, and develop personalised strategies to achieve your nutrition goals. Additionally, consider joining a support group or online community where you can connect with others who are also keeping food diaries and share tips, recipes, and encouragement.

Conclusion:

In conclusion, keeping a food diary is a valuable tool for improving your eating habits, managing your weight, and promoting overall health and well-being. By recording everything you eat and drink, including portion sizes and eating context, you can gain valuable insights into your dietary patterns and make informed choices about your nutrition. Whether you prefer pen and paper or a digital platform, consistency is key when it comes to keeping a food diary. Use your food diary as a tool for self-awareness, reflection, and improvement, and don't hesitate to seek support if needed. With dedication and commitment, keeping a food diary can help you achieve your health and wellness goals and live your best life.

MEASURING SUCCESS BEYOND THE SCALE

When it comes to health and wellness goals, such as weight loss or fitness improvement, many people tend to focus solely on the number on the scale. However, true success goes beyond just weight and encompasses a variety of factors that contribute to overall well-being. In this chapter, we'll explore practical tips for measuring success beyond the scale and shifting your focus to holistic health and wellness.

1. Define Your Definition of Success:

Before you can measure success beyond the scale, it's essential to define what success means to you personally. Take some time to reflect on your values, priorities, and goals, and consider what aspects of your life contribute to your overall happiness and well-being. Success may look different for everyone, whether it's feeling more energetic, improving your strength and endurance, or reducing stress and anxiety. By clarifying your definition of success, you can set meaningful goals and track your progress accordingly.

2. Focus on Non-Scale Victories:

Instead of solely relying on the number on the scale to measure your progress, celebrate non-scale victories that indicate improvements in your health and well-being. Non-scale victories can include things like:

- Increased energy levels
- Improved mood and mental clarity
- Better sleep quality
- Clothing fitting better or looser
- Increased strength and endurance
- Improved flexibility and mobility
- Reduced cravings for unhealthy foods
- Lower blood pressure or cholesterol levels
- Improved confidence and self-esteem

By shifting your focus to these non-scale victories, you'll gain a more holistic understanding of your progress and achievements, beyond just weight loss or gain.

3. Track Physical Fitness Progress:

Another valuable way to measure success beyond the scale is by tracking your physical fitness progress. Set specific fitness goals related to strength, endurance, flexibility, or athletic performance, and track your progress over time. Keep a workout log or journal to record your workouts, including exercises, sets, reps, and weights lifted. Use objective measures such as lifting heavier weights, running faster or farther, or mastering new yoga poses to gauge improvements in your fitness level. Celebrate milestones and achievements in your fitness journey, whether it's completing your first 5K race, mastering a challenging exercise, or achieving a personal best in the gym.

4. Assess Body Composition Changes:

Instead of fixating on the number on the scale, consider assessing changes in body composition to measure your progress more accurately. Body composition refers to the proportion of fat, muscle, bone, and water in your body, rather than just overall weight. Consider using other metrics such as body measurements (e.g., waist circumference, hip circumference, body fat percentage) or progress photos to track changes in your body composition over time. Remember that muscle weighs more than fat, so even if the scale doesn't budge, you may still be making positive changes to your body composition through exercise and healthy eating.

5. Monitor Health Markers:

Another important aspect of measuring success beyond the scale is monitoring key health markers that indicate improvements in your overall health and well-being. Consider tracking metrics such as blood pressure, cholesterol levels, blood sugar levels, resting heart rate, and other biomarkers that are relevant to your health goals. Regularly check in with your healthcare provider to assess your overall health and discuss any changes or improvements in your health markers. By focusing on improving these health markers, you can reduce your risk of chronic diseases and improve your long-term health outcomes.

6. Assess Mental and Emotional Well-Being:

In addition to physical health, it's essential to assess your mental and emotional well-being when measuring success beyond the scale. Pay attention to how you feel mentally and emotionally, including your mood, stress levels, anxiety levels, and overall sense of well-being. Consider incorporating stress management techniques such as mindfulness, meditation, deep breathing, or journaling into your daily routine to support your mental and emotional health. Seek support from a therapist or counsellor if you're struggling with mental health issues such as depression, anxiety, or disordered eating. Remember that mental and emotional well-being are just as important as physical health when it comes to overall well-being and quality of life.

7. Cultivate Healthy Habits:

Ultimately, success beyond the scale is about cultivating healthy habits that support your overall health and well-being. Focus on adopting sustainable lifestyle changes that promote physical, mental, and emotional health, rather than short-term fixes or fad diets. Prioritise habits such as regular exercise, balanced nutrition, adequate sleep, stress management, and social connection to support your holistic well-being. Celebrate small victories and progress along the way, and be patient with yourself as you work towards your goals. Remember that lasting change takes time and consistency, so focus on progress, not perfection, and celebrate the journey towards a healthier, happier you.

Conclusion:

In conclusion, measuring success beyond the scale involves looking beyond just weight and focusing on holistic health and well-being. By defining your definition of success, focusing on non-scale victories, tracking physical fitness progress, assessing body composition changes, monitoring health markers, assessing mental and emotional well-being, and cultivating healthy habits, you can gain a more comprehensive understanding of your progress and achievements. Remember that success is about more than just numbers on a scale; it's about feeling your best, inside and out, and living a life that aligns with your values and priorities. Embrace the journey towards holistic health and well-being, and celebrate the small victories along the way.

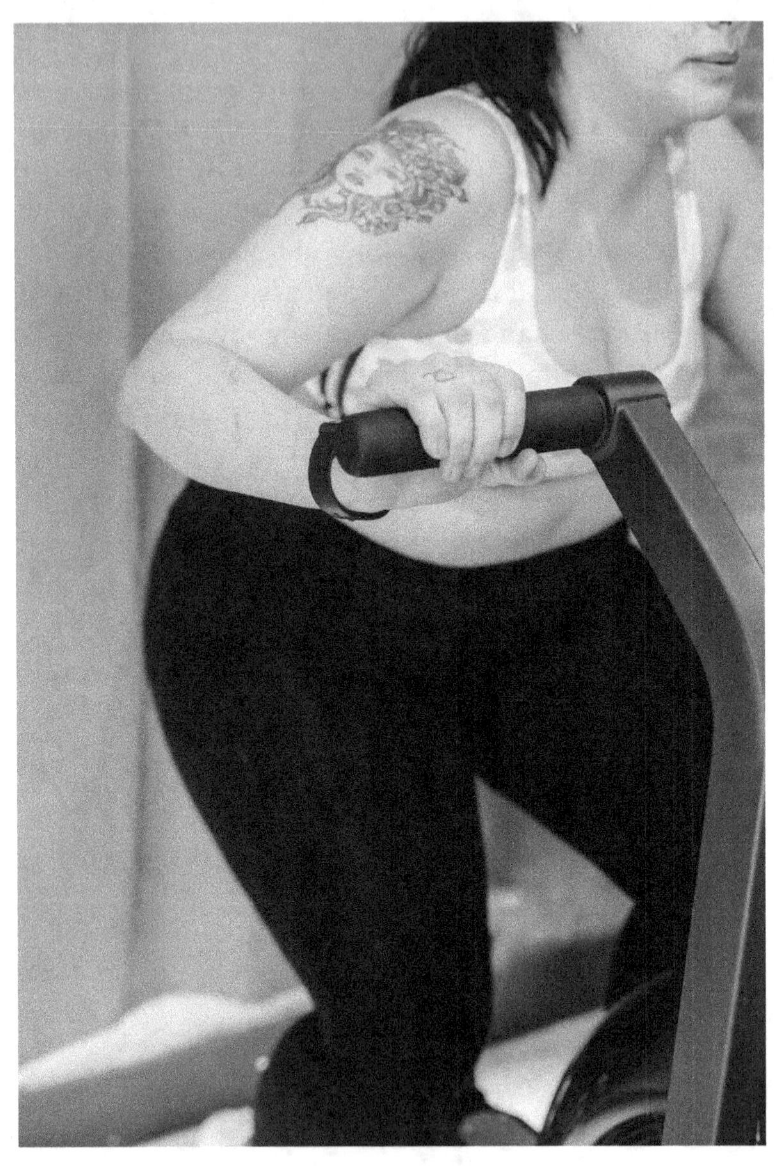

CHAPTER 11:
MAINTENANCE AND LONG -TERM SUCCESS

Achieving your health and wellness goals is a significant accomplishment, but maintaining your progress over the long term can be just as challenging. In this chapter, we'll explore the importance of maintenance and long-term success, and I'll share my personal experience to illustrate key points and strategies for sustaining your achievements.

Understanding Maintenance:

Maintenance is the phase of your journey where you transition from actively pursuing your goals to sustaining the progress you've made. It's about integrating healthy habits into your lifestyle and making them a permanent part of your routine. While the initial phase of goal attainment may involve significant effort and motivation, maintenance requires consistency, commitment, and resilience to overcome setbacks and challenges.

My Experience:

When I first embarked on my health and wellness journey, I was motivated and determined to make positive changes in my life. I set specific goals, developed a plan, and worked diligently to achieve them. However, as time passed, I realised that maintaining my progress was just as important as reaching my initial goals. I encountered setbacks and challenges along the way, but through trial and error, I learned valuable lessons about the importance of maintenance and long-term success.

Key Strategies for Maintenance:

1. Set Realistic Expectations:

One of the most crucial aspects of maintenance is setting realistic expectations for yourself. Recognize that progress may not always be linear, and setbacks are a natural part of the process. Be patient with yourself and focus on making gradual, sustainable changes rather than seeking quick fixes or drastic solutions. By setting realistic expectations, you'll set yourself up for long-term success and avoid feelings of frustration or disappointment.

2. Establish Healthy Habits:

To maintain your progress over the long term, focus on establishing healthy habits that support your goals. Whether it's regular exercise, balanced nutrition, adequate sleep, stress management, or self-care, prioritise habits that contribute to your overall health and well-being. Make these habits a non-negotiable part of your daily routine, and find ways to integrate them into your lifestyle seamlessly.

3. Practice Consistency:

Consistency is key when it comes to maintenance and long-term success. Stay committed to your goals and habits, even on days when motivation is low or obstacles arise. Remember that small, consistent actions add up over time and contribute to lasting change. Find strategies to stay accountable and motivated, whether it's tracking your progress, seeking support from others, or rewarding yourself for reaching milestones.

4. Be Flexible and Adaptive:

While consistency is essential, it's also important to be flexible and adaptive in your approach. Life is unpredictable, and you may encounter unexpected challenges or changes that require adjustments to your routine. Consider setbacks as opportunities to develop and learn rather than as failures. Be willing to adapt your strategies and make course corrections as needed to stay on track towards your goals.

5. Monitor Your Progress:

Regularly monitoring your progress is crucial for maintenance and long-term success. Keep track of key metrics, such as weight, body measurements, fitness level, and other relevant indicators, to assess your progress over time. Use this data to identify areas of improvement and make necessary adjustments to your approach. Celebrate your achievements and milestones along the way, and acknowledge the progress you've made, no matter how small.

6. Cultivate Resilience:

Maintaining long-term success requires resilience in the face of challenges and setbacks. Develop coping strategies to navigate obstacles, setbacks, and plateaus that may arise on your journey. Practice self-compassion and kindness towards yourself, and remember that setbacks are temporary and can be overcome with persistence and determination. Surround yourself with supportive people who believe in your ability to succeed and encourage you to keep going, even when the going gets tough.

7. Find Joy in the Journey:

Finally, remember to find joy in the journey towards maintenance and long-term success. Embrace the process of self-discovery, growth, and transformation, and celebrate the positive changes you've made in your life. Focus on the things that bring you happiness, fulfilment, and purpose, and cultivate a sense of gratitude for the progress you've achieved. By finding joy in the journey, you'll stay motivated, inspired, and committed to sustaining your achievements for years to come.

Conclusion:

In conclusion, maintenance and long-term success are essential components of any health and wellness journey. By setting realistic expectations, establishing healthy habits, practising consistency, being flexible and adaptive, monitoring your progress, cultivating resilience, and finding joy in the journey, you can sustain your achievements and continue to thrive over the long term. Remember that maintenance is not a destination but a lifelong process, and embrace the opportunity to live your best life every day.

STRATEGIES FOR MAINTAINING WEIGHT LOSS

While losing weight is a great accomplishment, keeping the weight off in the long run is more difficult. Many people struggle with regaining lost weight after reaching their goal, but with the right strategies in place, it's possible to sustain your weight loss and enjoy a healthier, happier life. In this chapter, we'll explore practical tips for maintaining weight loss and preventing regain.

1. Focus on Sustainable Lifestyle Changes:

The key to maintaining weight loss is adopting sustainable lifestyle changes that you can maintain over the long term. Instead of relying on fad diets or quick-fix solutions, focus on making gradual, sustainable changes to your eating habits, physical activity, and overall lifestyle. Choose nutritious, whole foods, prioritise regular exercise, get adequate sleep, manage stress effectively, and practice self-care. By building healthy habits into your daily routine, you'll create a solid foundation for long-term success.

2. Eat Mindfully:

Mindful eating is a powerful tool for maintaining weight loss and preventing overeating. Eat gently, pay attention to your hunger and fullness signs, and enjoy every bite. Be mindful of portion sizes, and avoid distractions such as television, smartphones, or computers while eating. Focus on the taste, texture, and satisfaction of your food, and stop eating when you feel comfortably full. By practising mindful eating, you'll develop a healthier relationship with food and become more in tune with your body's needs.

3. Monitor Your Eating Habits:

Regularly monitoring your eating habits can help you stay on track and identify potential triggers for overeating or unhealthy behaviours. Keep a food diary or use a food tracking app to record your meals, snacks, and beverages, as well as your emotions, cravings, and eating patterns. Look for patterns or trends in your eating habits, such as emotional eating, mindless snacking, or eating out of boredom, and develop strategies to address these behaviours. By staying aware of your eating habits, you can make informed choices and prevent mindless eating.

4. Stay Active:

Regular physical activity is essential for maintaining weight loss and supporting overall health and well-being. Aim for 75 minutes of strenuous activity or at least 150 minutes of moderate-intensity aerobic activity per week, in addition to two or more days of muscle-strengthening activities. Find activities that you enjoy and can incorporate into your daily routine, such as walking, cycling, swimming, or dancing. Stay active throughout the day by taking the stairs instead of the elevator, walking or biking instead of driving, and incorporating movement breaks into your day. By staying active, you'll burn calories, boost your metabolism, and maintain muscle mass, making it easier to sustain your weight loss over time.

5. Plan and Prepare Meals:

Meal planning and preparation are essential for maintaining weight loss and preventing impulsive eating or unhealthy food choices. Take the time to plan your meals and snacks for the week ahead, and prepare healthy, balanced meals in advance. Stock your kitchen with nutritious ingredients, such as fruits, vegetables, lean proteins, whole grains, and healthy fats, and avoid keeping tempting or unhealthy foods in the house. Batch cook and portion out meals and snacks to make healthy eating more convenient and accessible throughout the week. By planning and preparing meals ahead of time, you'll be less likely to rely on fast food or takeout and more likely to make nourishing choices that support your weight loss goals.

6. Practice Self-Care:

Self-care is an essential component of maintaining weight loss and promoting overall well-being. Take time for yourself each day to relax, unwind, and recharge your batteries. Engage in activities that bring you joy and fulfilment, such as reading, meditating, spending time outdoors, or pursuing hobbies and interests. Prioritise sleep and aim for seven to nine hours of quality sleep each night to support your physical and mental health. Manage stress effectively through relaxation techniques such as deep breathing, meditation, yoga, or tai chi. By prioritising self-care, you'll reduce your risk of emotional eating, improve your mood and energy levels, and maintain a healthy balance in your life.

7. Seek Support:

Maintaining weight loss can be challenging, but you don't have to do it alone. Seek support from friends, family members, or a support group who can offer encouragement, accountability, and practical advice. Consider working with a registered dietitian, nutritionist, or health coach who can provide personalised guidance and support to help you stay on track. Join an online community or forum where you can connect with others who are also working towards weight maintenance goals and share tips, strategies, and success stories. By surrounding yourself with supportive people who understand your journey, you'll be more likely to stay motivated and committed to maintaining your weight loss over the long term.

Conclusion:

In conclusion, maintaining weight loss requires a commitment to sustainable lifestyle changes, mindful eating, regular physical activity, meal planning and preparation, self-care, and seeking support from others. By incorporating these strategies into your daily routine, you can sustain your weight loss and enjoy a healthier, happier life for years to come. Remember that maintaining weight loss is a journey, not a destination, and be patient with yourself as you navigate the ups and downs along the way. With dedication, consistency, and support, you can achieve long-term success and maintain your weight loss goals for life.

BUILDING HEALTHY HABITS FOR LIFE

Building healthy habits is essential for promoting overall well-being and longevity. Whether you're looking to improve your physical health, mental well-being, or overall quality of life, adopting healthy habits can help you achieve your goals and sustain them for the long term. In this chapter, we'll explore practical tips for building healthy habits that you can incorporate into your daily routine.

1. Start Small:

Establishing healthy habits requires tiny steps at first. Instead of trying to overhaul your entire lifestyle overnight, focus on making small, manageable changes that you can sustain over time. Choose one or two habits to work on initially, such as drinking more water, eating an extra serving of vegetables each day, or going for a short walk after dinner. Once you've mastered these habits, you can gradually add more to your repertoire.

2. Set Specific Goals:

To build healthy habits effectively, it's important to set specific, measurable goals that you can work towards. Instead of setting vague goals like "eat healthier" or "exercise more," be specific about what you want to achieve and establish clear criteria for success. For example, set a goal to eat five servings of fruits and vegetables per day or to walk for 30 minutes five days a week. Having concrete goals gives you something to aim for and helps keep you motivated and accountable.

3. Make It Convenient:

One of the most effective ways to build healthy habits is to make them as convenient as possible. Identify barriers or obstacles that may be preventing you from adopting healthy habits and find ways to overcome them. For example, if you struggle to find time to exercise, schedule workouts into your calendar and treat them like appointments. If you find it challenging to eat healthy meals at home, consider meal prepping or batch cooking on weekends to have healthy options readily available during the week.

4. Focus on Consistency:

Establishing good behaviours requires consistency. Make a commitment to practise your chosen habits consistently, even on days when you don't feel like it or when life gets busy. Aim for progress, not perfection, and focus on showing up and putting in effort each day. Over time, consistent practice will help solidify your habits and make them feel like second nature.

5. Find What Works for You:

There's no one-size-fits-all approach to building healthy habits, so it's essential to find what works best for you. Experiment with different strategies, techniques, and routines to see what resonates with you and fits your lifestyle. If you enjoy group exercise classes, make that a regular part of your routine. If you prefer to exercise outdoors, find activities like hiking, biking, or jogging that you enjoy. Likewise, if you struggle to cook at home, explore options like meal delivery services or healthy takeout options that align with your goals.

6. Practice Mindfulness:

Mindfulness is a powerful tool for building healthy habits and promoting overall well-being. By practising mindfulness, you can become more aware of your thoughts, feelings, and behaviours related to health and wellness. Pay attention to your body's hunger and fullness cues, notice how different foods make you feel, and be mindful of the choices you make throughout the day. Mindfulness can help you break free from automatic or unhealthy habits and make more intentional choices that support your well-being.

7. Seek Support:

Building healthy habits is often easier when you have support from others. Share your goals and aspirations with friends, family members, or a supportive community who can offer encouragement, accountability, and practical advice. Consider partnering with a workout buddy, joining a fitness class, or participating in a group challenge to stay motivated and inspired. Surround yourself with people who share your values and goals and who can help you stay on track when the going gets tough.

8. Be Patient and Persistent:

Building healthy habits takes time, patience, and persistence. Don't expect to see overnight results, and be prepared to encounter setbacks and challenges along the way. Rather of letting failures depress you, see them as chances for development and education. Be kind to yourself, celebrate your progress, and keep moving forward, even when progress feels slow or difficult. Remember that building healthy habits is a journey, not a destination, and every small step you take brings you closer to your goals.

Conclusion:

In conclusion, building healthy habits is essential for promoting overall well-being and longevity. By starting small, setting specific goals, making habits convenient, focusing on consistency, finding what works for you, practicing mindfulness, seeking support, and being patient and persistent, you can build healthy habits that last a lifetime. Remember that building healthy habits is a gradual process, so be patient with yourself and celebrate your progress along the way. With dedication, commitment, and a willingness to experiment, you can create a healthier life for yourself.

CELEBRATING MILESTONES AND ACHIEVEMENTS

In the journey of life, it's important to pause and acknowledge our accomplishments along the way. Whether big or small, milestones and achievements are worth celebrating as they represent progress, growth, and success. In this chapter, we'll explore the significance of celebrating milestones and achievements and provide practical tips on how to do so in a meaningful and rewarding way.

1. Recognize the Importance:

Celebrating milestones and achievements is more than just a moment of joy; it's an essential part of the journey towards our goals. By taking the time to acknowledge our progress and successes, we reinforce positive behaviours, boost our confidence, and stay motivated to continue working towards our aspirations. Additionally, celebrating milestones allows us to reflect on how far we've come and appreciate the hard work and effort we've invested along the way.

2. Set Clear Milestones:

To effectively celebrate milestones and achievements, it's crucial to set clear and measurable goals along the way. Break down your larger goals into smaller, achievable milestones that you can celebrate as you progress. For example, if your goal is to run a marathon, your milestones could include completing a certain distance in training, achieving a new personal best in a race, or reaching a specific number of training sessions. Having clear milestones gives you something to strive for and provides opportunities for celebration throughout your journey.

3. Choose Meaningful Rewards:

When celebrating milestones and achievements, consider choosing rewards that are meaningful and aligned with your goals. Instead of resorting to material rewards or indulgent treats, think about ways to reward yourself that reinforce positive behaviours and contribute to your overall well-being. For example, if you've reached a fitness milestone, reward yourself with a relaxing massage, a new workout outfit, or a day of rest and recovery. If you've achieved a career milestone, celebrate by treating yourself to a professional development course, a mentorship opportunity, or a networking event. By choosing rewards that align with your values and goals, you'll reinforce positive habits and stay motivated to continue making progress.

4. Share Your Success:

Celebrating milestones and achievements is even more meaningful when shared with others. Don't hesitate to share your successes with friends, family members, colleagues, or your community who can offer support, encouragement, and congratulations. Share your journey on social media, write a blog post, or send out a newsletter to update others on your progress and accomplishments. Not only does sharing your success allow you to bask in the glow of your achievements, but it also inspires others to pursue their goals and celebrate their own milestones along the way.

5. Reflect and Appreciate:

In the midst of celebrating milestones and achievements, take time to reflect on your journey and appreciate the lessons learned along the way. Reflect on the challenges you've overcome, the obstacles you've faced, and the growth and personal development you've experienced. Take stock of the skills, strengths, and qualities that have contributed to your success and express gratitude for the support and encouragement you've received from others. By reflecting on your journey and appreciating your accomplishments, you'll gain a deeper sense of fulfilment and motivation to continue striving towards your goals.

6. Cultivate a Growth Mindset:

When celebrating milestones and achievements, it's important to cultivate a growth mindset that focuses on progress, learning, and improvement. Instead of viewing success as a destination, see it as a journey of continuous growth and development. Embrace challenges as opportunities for growth, learn from setbacks and failures, and celebrate progress, no matter how small. By adopting a growth mindset, you'll stay resilient in the face of obstacles, maintain a positive outlook, and continue making strides towards your goals.

7. Create Rituals and Traditions:

To make celebrating milestones and achievements a regular part of your routine, consider creating rituals and traditions that mark significant moments along your journey. Whether it's ringing a bell, lighting a candle, or sharing a meal with loved ones, find rituals that hold meaning for you and incorporate them into your celebrations. These rituals can serve as reminders of your progress and accomplishments and provide a sense of continuity and connection throughout your journey.

Conclusion:

In conclusion, celebrating milestones and achievements is an essential part of the journey towards our goals. By recognizing the importance of celebrating milestones, setting clear goals, choosing meaningful rewards, sharing our success, reflecting and appreciating, cultivating a growth mindset, and creating rituals and traditions, we can make celebrating our accomplishments a meaningful and rewarding experience. Remember to celebrate not only the destination but also the journey, and take time to acknowledge and appreciate the progress you've made along the way. With each milestone celebrated, we reinforce positive behaviours, boost our confidence, and stay motivated to continue pursuing our dreams and aspirations.

CONCLUSION :
WEIGHT LOSS FOR WOMEN OVER 45

In conclusion, embarking on a weight loss journey for women over 45 can be both challenging and rewarding. As we age, our bodies undergo various changes, including hormonal shifts, metabolic slowdown, and changes in muscle mass, which can make it more difficult to lose weight and keep it off. However, with dedication, commitment, and the right strategies in place, women over 45 can achieve their weight loss goals and enjoy improved health and well-being.

Throughout this guide, we've explored various factors that impact weight loss for women over 45, including metabolism, hormonal changes, dietary considerations, exercise strategies, mindset shifts, and lifestyle modifications. We've also provided practical tips and actionable advice to help women over 45 navigate the challenges of weight loss and create sustainable habits for long-term success.

Here are some key takeaways and practical tips for women over 45 to consider as they continue their weight loss journey:

1. Prioritise Nutrition: Focus on nourishing your body with nutrient-dense foods that support overall health and well-being. Choose a balanced diet rich in fruits, vegetables, lean proteins, whole grains, and healthy fats. To prevent overeating, be attentive of portion sizes and engage in mindful eating.

2. Stay Active: Incorporate regular physical activity into your routine to support weight loss and improve overall fitness. Aim for a combination of aerobic exercise, strength training, flexibility, and balance exercises to promote overall health and well-being. Make time for the things you enjoy doing on a regular basis.

3. Manage Stress: Chronic stress can contribute to weight gain and make it harder to lose weight, especially for women over 45. Practice stress management techniques such as deep breathing, meditation, yoga, or tai chi to reduce stress levels and promote relaxation. Make time for self-care activities that will allow you to relax and rejuvenate.

4. Get Adequate Sleep: Lack of sleep can disrupt hormonal balance, increase appetite, and sabotage weight loss efforts. Aim for seven to nine hours of

quality sleep each night to support weight loss and overall health. To encourage sound sleep, establish a nightly ritual and make your surroundings conducive to relaxation.

5. Seek Support: Encircle yourself with a network of friends, family, or a qualified coach who can provide accountability, inspiration, and useful guidance. Join a weight loss group, participate in online forums, or seek guidance from a registered dietitian or nutritionist who specialises in weight loss for women over 45.

6. Set Realistic Goals: Set realistic and achievable goals for weight loss, taking into account factors such as age, metabolism, and lifestyle. Prioritise development over perfection and acknowledge even the smallest accomplishments along the route. Be patient with yourself and recognize that sustainable weight loss takes time and effort.

7. Focus on Health, Not Just Weight: Instead of fixating solely on the number on the scale, focus on improving overall health and well-being. Monitor other markers of health such as blood pressure, cholesterol levels, blood sugar, energy levels, and mood. Celebrate improvements in these areas as signs of progress, regardless of changes in weight.

8. Stay Consistent: Consistency is key when it comes to successful weight loss for women over 45. Stick to your healthy eating and exercise habits consistently, even on days when motivation is low or obstacles arise. Remember that small, consistent actions add up over time and contribute to long-term success.

In summary, weight loss for women over 45 is achievable with the right mindset, strategies, and support system in place. By prioritising nutrition, staying active, managing stress, getting adequate sleep, seeking support, setting realistic goals, focusing on health, and staying consistent, women over 45 can achieve their weight loss goals and enjoy improved health and well-being. Remember that every step forward, no matter how small, brings you closer to your goals, and celebrate your progress along the way. With dedication and perseverance, you can create a healthier, happier life for yourself at any age.

Final Thoughts

As we come to the end of this guide, I'm reminded of the journey we've embarked on together – a journey of self-discovery, growth, and transformation. Throughout these pages, we've explored various aspects of health, wellness, and personal development, delving into topics ranging from weight loss and healthy habits to mindset shifts and goal setting. As we wrap up our discussion, I'd like to share some final thoughts and reflections, drawing from both the insights shared in this guide and my own personal experience.

1. Embrace the Journey:

Life is a journey, not a destination, and the same holds true for our health and wellness goals. Instead of focusing solely on the end result, embrace the process of growth and transformation that occurs along the way. Every setback, challenge, and triumph is an opportunity for learning and growth. Embrace the journey, celebrate the small victories, and keep moving forward with determination and resilience.

2. Cultivate Self-Compassion:

In our pursuit of health and wellness, it's essential to practise self-compassion and kindness towards ourselves. Be gentle with yourself on this journey, and remember that progress is not always linear. It's okay to stumble, to make mistakes, and to have setbacks. What's important is how we respond to these challenges with kindness, understanding, and self-love. Treat yourself with the same kindness and compassion that you would offer to a dear friend.

3. Stay Open-Minded:

As we navigate the ever-changing landscape of health and wellness, it's important to stay open-minded and curious. Be willing to explore new ideas, perspectives, and approaches to health and well-being. What works for one person may not work for another, so be open to experimenting and finding what resonates with you personally. Stay curious, ask questions, and remain open to the possibility of growth and transformation.

4. Practice Gratitude:

Gratitude is a powerful practice that can help shift our perspective and cultivate a sense of abundance in our lives. Take a moment each day to reflect on the things you're grateful for – whether it's your health, your loved ones, or simply the beauty of nature around you. By focusing on the blessings in your life, you'll cultivate a positive mindset and attract more positivity into your life.

5. Keep Moving Forward:

No matter where you are on your health and wellness journey, remember that progress is progress, no matter how small. Keep moving forward, one step at a time, and trust in the process. Setbacks and obstacles are inevitable, but it's how we respond to them that ultimately determines our success. Stay focused on your goals, stay committed to your vision, and never lose sight of the incredible potential within you.

6. Find Joy in the Process:

Above all, remember to find joy in the process of self-improvement and personal growth. Life is too short to spend it obsessing over the number on the scale or chasing after perfection. Instead, focus on nourishing your body, nurturing your soul, and living life to the fullest. Find joy in the simple pleasures – a walk in nature, a nutritious meal shared with loved ones, or a quiet moment of reflection. By finding joy in the process, you'll cultivate a deeper sense of fulfilment and contentment in your life.

In conclusion, I hope this guide has provided you with valuable insights, practical tips, and inspiration to embark on your own journey towards health, wellness, and personal growth. Remember that you are capable of achieving incredible things, and that your journey is uniquely yours. Embrace the challenges, celebrate the victories, and above all, never stop believing in yourself. Here's to a lifetime of health, happiness, and fulfilment.

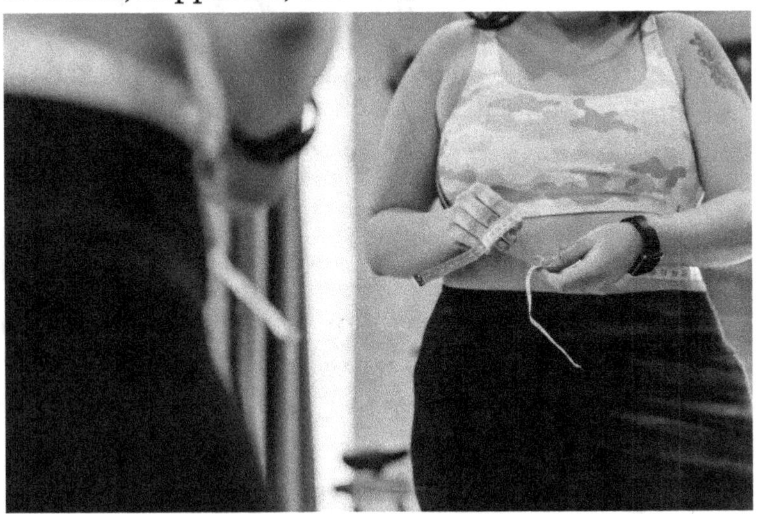

ENCOURAGEMENT FOR CONTINUED SUCCESS

Congratulations on taking steps towards achieving your goals and making positive changes in your life! As you continue on your journey towards success, it's important to stay motivated, focused, and resilient. In this chapter, we'll explore practical tips and words of encouragement to help you stay on track and continue moving forward towards your goals.

1. Reflect on Your Progress:

Take a moment to reflect on how far you've come since you first started your journey. Celebrate the progress you've made, no matter how small, and acknowledge the hard work and dedication it took to get to where you are today. Reflecting on your achievements can help boost your confidence, reignite your motivation, and remind you of your capability to overcome obstacles and achieve your goals.

2. Set New Goals:

As you reach milestones and achieve success, it's important to continue setting new goals to keep yourself challenged and motivated. Consider where you want to be in the next month, six months, or year, and set clear, actionable goals to work towards. Whether it's improving your fitness level, learning a new skill, or pursuing a passion project, setting new goals will keep you focused and driven on your journey towards continued success.

3. Find Inspiration:

Surround yourself with sources of inspiration that motivate and uplift you. Seek out stories of individuals who have achieved success in areas that resonate with you, whether it's health and fitness, career advancement, personal development, or creative pursuits. Follow inspiring figures on social media, read books or articles that inspire you, and connect with like-minded individuals who share your goals and aspirations. Drawing inspiration from others can help fuel your own journey towards success.

4. Practice Self-Care:

Taking care of yourself is essential for maintaining the energy, motivation, and resilience needed to pursue your goals. Make self-care a priority by prioritizing activities that nourish your body, mind, and soul. This may include getting adequate sleep, eating nutritious meals, exercising regularly, practicing mindfulness or meditation, spending time in nature, or engaging in activities that bring you joy and relaxation. By taking care of yourself, you'll be better equipped to handle challenges and stay focused on your path to success.

5. Stay Positive:

Maintaining a positive mindset is crucial for overcoming obstacles and staying motivated on your journey towards success. Focus on cultivating a positive outlook by practising gratitude, reframing negative thoughts, and surrounding yourself with positivity. When faced with challenges or setbacks, remind yourself of your past successes and the resilience you've demonstrated in overcoming obstacles. Believe in your ability to overcome challenges and achieve your goals, and approach each day with optimism and determination.

6. Seek Support:

Don't hesitate to reach out for support from friends, family members, mentors, or a supportive community who can offer encouragement, guidance, and accountability. Share your goals and aspirations with others who can provide support and cheer you on as you work towards success. Consider joining a mastermind group, participating in online forums or support groups, or seeking guidance from a coach or mentor who can provide personalised support and guidance on your journey.

7. Stay Flexible:

While it's important to stay focused on your goals, it's also important to stay flexible and adaptable in the face of change and uncertainty. Recognize that setbacks and obstacles are a natural part of the journey towards success, and be willing to adjust your plans and strategies as needed. Stay open to new opportunities, be willing to learn from your experiences, and embrace the unexpected twists and turns that come your way. By staying flexible, you'll be better equipped to navigate challenges and stay on course towards your goals.

8. Celebrate Your Achievements:

Lastly, remember to recognize and honour your progress along the road. Take time to acknowledge and celebrate your successes, no matter how small, and recognize the progress you've made towards your goals. Whether it's treating yourself to a special reward, sharing your achievements with loved ones, or simply taking a moment to reflect and appreciate your accomplishments, celebrating your successes will boost your confidence, motivation, and sense of accomplishment.

In conclusion, remember that success is a journey, not a destination, and staying motivated and focused is essential for continued success. By reflecting on your progress, setting new goals, finding inspiration, practising self-care, staying positive, seeking support, staying flexible, and celebrating your achievements, you'll stay on track towards your goals and keep accomplishing success in every aspect of your life. Never give up, maintain your fortitude, and never lose sight of the amazing potential you possess. You've got this!